FROM OBESITY TO WELLNESS

The Ultimate Guide to Lifestyle Medicine for Obesity
Management, Offering a Blend of Science, Practicality, and
Compassion for Optimum Health

By: Dr. Grace Totoe

11/10/24

To wellness and hope

Dedication

To David, Maia, and Ava—my family, my everything. You ground me in ways words can hardly capture. Your support, love, and laughter are my guiding lights, illuminating my path in this world.

This book is for you. It's a celebration of the love we share and a testament to the power of family. May it inspire those who read it to hold their loved ones close, just as I hold you.

Supporting Health Equity

By purchasing this book, you're not just gaining a guide to better health but also contributing to a more significant cause. A portion of the proceeds from this book will be dedicated to supporting health equity in the United States and Africa, focusing on providing healthcare to marginalized communities. Your support helps us extend our reach and impact through the work of the **"Totoe Health Equity Project."**

Learn more about our mission and how you can further contribute at www.totoe-equity.com. Together, we can make a difference in the lives of those in need.

Table of Contents

Introduction

"Health is not just the absence of disease; it's the harmony of the body, mind, and spirit. Caring for our bodies nurtures our souls and strengthens our minds. The journey to wellness begins with a single step towards understanding and embracing a life of balance."

In my years of practice as a medical physician and lifestyle advocate, I've encountered many stories, each unique and deeply personal. But one story that resonates with me, and perhaps will with you too, is that of Susan, an African mother of four. Her journey is not just a tale of struggle with weight but a testament to the resilience and challenges so many face daily.

I met Susan during one of my routine clinic visits. The first thing you'd notice about her was her infectious smile, which sadly concealed more than it revealed. Susan juggled a full-time job and a catering business, a testament to her incredible work ethic and dedication. But that's just the tip of the iceberg. After her day job, she transformed into a supermom – shuttling her kids to basketball and various activities, ensuring everyone was fed, and the kitchen spotless before she could even think of resting.

Over the years, amidst the chaos of life and her ceaseless dedication to her family, Susan's health took a backseat. She had gained about 120 pounds through her four pregnancies. Like many, she tried to regain control – intermittent fasting, healthy eating – but stress often derailed her efforts, leading to periodic overeating. Now, tipping the scales at 260 pounds, her body constantly reminded her of the burden it bore. Her hips, knees, and lower back ached incessantly, a silent cry for help from her weary frame.

But the physical pain wasn't the only thing weighing her down. Susan's vibrant social life had dwindled, not just due to her hectic schedule but also because of the shame and embarrassment she felt about her appearance. The stark contrast between her current self and the basketball star she once was in high school made her avoid reunions and social gatherings. The thought of facing her former teammates, who remembered her in her athletic prime, was too much to bear.

One quiet evening, as she sat alone, the walls of her home echoing the silence of her thoughts, Susan arrived at a crossroads. It was a moment of profound realization – she couldn't let life continue to pass her by. She deserved more than this cycle of neglect and unfulfilled potential. That night, Susan made a decision that would not only change her life but also pave the way for physical and emotional healing.

Why am I sharing this with you? This story isn't just Susan's; it reflects the journey of many. It's a narrative that resonates across continents, in bustling cities and quiet towns, among individuals from all walks of life. Obesity is not just a personal challenge; it's a global epidemic that touches the lives of billions. It doesn't discriminate, affecting the young and old, the busy professionals and the stay-at-home parents, the physically active and those less so. Susan's story is a mirror, reflecting the struggles of countless others who find themselves in a similar battle against weight and its accompanying hardships.

It's crucial to understand the magnitude of this issue. According to the World Health Organization, more than 1 billion people worldwide are obese. This staggering figure includes 650 million adults, 340 million adolescents, and 39 million children. And the numbers are rising. By 2025, WHO estimates that approximately 167 million people, both adults and children, will suffer from health issues directly linked to being overweight or obese. These aren't just numbers; they're individuals with stories, families, dreams, and struggles. They are people like Susan who confront the daily realities of obesity.

This book aims to shed light on these realities, offering not just guidance and understanding but also practical, tangible solutions. It's not simply about shedding pounds; it's about embracing a holistic journey towards wellness. Lifestyle medicine, a cornerstone of this journey, is an empowering approach that integrates nutrition, stress management, quality sleep, and regular exercise. Each component plays a crucial role in combating obesity and enhancing overall health. I'm here to help you navigate these elements, make informed and transformative choices, and understand your body in ways you might never have considered before.

Together, we'll embark on a journey that goes beyond the surface. We'll have a full understanding of obesity, examining its various causes and far-reaching health implications. But more than that, we'll address the psychological battles that often go hand-in-hand with this condition. The comprehensive approach extends beyond dieting and physical activity. We're talking about a shift in mindset, a new way to perceive and interact with your health and lifestyle.

Susan's decision to seek help was a turning point in her life. It's the kind of decision I hope to inspire in you through this book. Her story is a starting point, a catalyst for change. As we journey through these pages together, I aim to guide, support, and empower you, just as Susan was, on your path from obesity to wellness.

Chapter 1: Understanding Obesity

"Obesity is not about the weight you carry, but the weight that carries you. It's a personal story written in the language of the body."

When we talk about obesity, what exactly comes to your mind? Is it merely about being significantly overweight, or do you also consider other factors? Well, it's time to dive a little deeper and understand the full scope of this condition.

Obesity isn't just a number on a scale; it's a medical condition characterized by excessive body fat. But how much is too much, and what does that look like for different people? That's where the Body Mass Index (BMI) comes into play. BMI is a tool that uses your height and weight to estimate how much body fat you have. Generally, a BMI of 30 or higher is considered obese.

To calculate your BMI, simply use this formula:

$$BMI = \text{weight in kilograms} / (\text{height in meters})^2$$

Or, for those using pounds and inches:

$$BMI = (\text{weight in pounds} / (\text{height in inches})^2 \times 703$$

Now, it's important to remember that BMI isn't the whole story. It doesn't differentiate between fat and muscle, nor does it account for where fat is on your body. Doctors often use it as a starting point, not a diagnostic endpoint.

But why does this distinction matter? Because obesity isn't just about appearance. It's a health issue that can have serious implications. It affects almost every part of your body, from your bones to your heart and digestive system to your brain. Understanding obesity is the first step in recognizing its impact on your life and taking control of your health journey.

Now, let's take a moment and explore your perceptions and beliefs around obesity. Reflecting on these questions not only enhances your understanding but also prepares you to engage more empathetically and knowledgeably on this topic.

QUICK Reflection:

- How does your understanding of obesity change when considering it beyond just a number on the scale?
- Reflect on any misconceptions you might have had about BMI and its effectiveness in truly capturing health.

Now, take a moment to write down three ways you think society's perception of obesity could be more compassionate and informed.

The Root Causes: Genetic, Lifestyle, and Environmental Factors

U nderstanding obesity also means exploring why it happens. It's like a puzzle with many pieces, and these pieces are different for everyone – has three leading players: *genetics, lifestyle, and the environment.*

First, let's talk about genetics. Our genes play a role in determining our body weight. They affect appetite, metabolism, and how our bodies store fat. But it's not a simple one-to-one relationship. Think of your genetic makeup as a blueprint. It sets the stage, but it's only part of the story. Your lifestyle choices and environment interact with this blueprint, shaping the final outcome.

Lifestyle factors are our daily choices – what we eat, how active we are, and our sleeping patterns. A diet high in calories, lack of physical activity, and inadequate sleep can all contribute to weight gain. It's like a domino effect; one unhealthy choice can set off a chain reaction leading to obesity.

Then there's the environment, which encompasses everything from your social circle to your workplace habits, from the availability of healthy food options to the walkability of your neighborhood. Our environment can either support healthy choices or make them more challenging.

So, obesity isn't just about willpower. It's about how these factors interact. Understanding this can help us be more compassionate towards ourselves and others in the journey to better health.

Reflection:

Identify one lifestyle factor and one environmental factor in your life that might be influencing your health. How can you address these factors?

- **Exercise:**

Create a simple plan to incorporate more physical activity into your week. Consider your current environment and how it can support or hinder this plan.

Health Implications of Obesity

The impact of obesity extends far beyond the number you see on the scale, affecting nearly every system in your body in profound ways. This isn't just about weight; it's a complex interplay of health issues that affects your body system and overall well-being.

Cardiovascular System:
When we think of obesity, the heart often comes to mind first, and rightly so. Excess weight has been linked with increased risks of heart disease and stroke. The extra weight doesn't just sit; it strains the heart, escalating the chances of high blood pressure, cholesterol issues, and atherosclerosis. These conditions can lead to heart attacks, heart failure, and even decreased blood supply to vital organs, posing a threat to life itself.

Respiratory System:
Your lungs, too, feel the weight of obesity. The excessive fat in the chest and abdomen can hinder lung expansion, leading to breathing difficulties. This raises the risk of sleep apnea, asthma, and even pulmonary hypertension – a condition that can lead to life-threatening blood clots.

Metabolic System:
Then there's the tie between obesity and metabolic disorders. Excess fat can disrupt insulin function, reducing its sensitivity, spiking blood sugar levels and heightening the risk of type 2 diabetes. This not only affects your blood sugar but also loops back to exacerbating heart problems.

Musculoskeletal System:
Our bones and joints bear the literal burden of excess weight. Obesity heightens the risk of osteoarthritis, particularly in the knees and hips. This can spiral into chronic pain, reduced mobility, and even an increased risk of fractures and related complications like blood clots and chronic pain management issues.

Gastrointestinal System:

Digestive issues also arise with obesity. From acid reflux to gallbladder disease and fatty liver disease, the risk of inflammation and scarring in the liver can progress to cirrhosis, which carries a high mortality rate and is often complicated by infections and other severe medical challenges.

Mental Health:
We cannot overlook the mental and emotional toll of obesity. Depression, anxiety, low self-esteem, and body image issues are common. The social stigma and discrimination can exacerbate psychological distress, potentially leading to more severe conditions like severe depression and even suicidal tendencies.

Obesity, therefore, is not a standalone issue. It's a mixture of health concerns, each impacting and exacerbating the other. Addressing obesity requires acknowledging its complexity and adopting a multi–disciplinary approach considering dietary, physical, behavioral, and sometimes medical interventions. It's about seeing the full picture, understanding the varied impacts, and taking a holistic step toward healing and wellness.

Now, reflect on how understanding the broader health implications of obesity changes the way you view the condition. Is it more serious or complex than you initially thought?

- **Exercise for you:**

Consider any health symptoms you experience. Could they be related to weight? How might addressing weight impact these conditions?

Debunking Myths: Separating Fact from Fiction in Obesity

In our quest to understand obesity, it's crucial to dismantle some common myths that cloud our perception of this condition. Let's set the record straight and replace misconceptions with facts:

1. Myth of Personal Choice and Laziness:
It's easy to think that obesity is just about personal choices or a lack of activity. But the truth is far more complex. Obesity intertwines genetic, environmental, and behavioral factors. It's not a simple matter of willpower. Genetics, metabolism, socioeconomic status, chronic pain, mental health, medications, and even access to healthy food options play significant roles in influencing one's weight.

2. Myth of Weight as the Sole Health Indicator:
Often, we equate health solely with weight. While obesity does increase the risk of various health issues, being thin doesn't automatically mean being healthy. Health is a broader concept involving diet, physical activity, and other lifestyle factors. True health assessment should encompass the overall lifestyle, not just the scale.

3. Myth of Willpower in Weight Loss:
"Just eat less and move more, and you'll lose weight." If only it were that simple! Weight loss is a journey that requires more than willpower. It involves diet, exercise, behavior changes, and sometimes even medical interventions. It's a multifaceted challenge, demanding a comprehensive and personalized approach.

4. Myth of Calorie Intake as the Sole Cause:
The idea that obesity is just about eating too much is a narrow view. Yes, calorie intake matters, but so do hormonal imbalances, genetics, certain medications, stress levels, and sleep patterns.

Obesity is not a one-cause issue; it's a complex interplay of various factors.

5. Myth of Weight Loss as the Only Goal:
Fixating on weight loss alone can be a narrow approach to obesity. It's not just about shedding pounds; it's about overall health improvement. Reducing obesity-related disease risks and enhancing quality of life are equally important. A holistic view focuses on health, not just the number on the scale.

6. Myth of 'One-Size-Fits-All' Solutions:
There's a common belief that what works for one person will work for everyone. But when it comes to obesity, each journey is unique. Individual differences in body chemistry, lifestyle, and psychology mean that what's effective for one person may not be for another. Personalized approaches are key.

7. Myth of Obesity as a Purely Physical Condition:
Often, we view obesity only through a physical lens. However, it's also deeply intertwined with emotional and mental health. Stress, emotional well-being, and self-image play crucial roles in managing obesity. Understanding this can foster a more compassionate and comprehensive approach to treatment.

It's important to understand the real facts about obesity. There are many misconceptions out there that can make it harder for people to get the help they need. By learning the truth, we can be more understanding and effective in helping people manage their weight. Everyone faces different challenges when it comes to staying healthy, so it's important to be open to other strategies and approaches.

Chapter thoughts:

As we wrap up the first chapter, which delves into the essentials of understanding obesity, let's pause for a moment of reflection. This chapter aimed not only to inform but to challenge and expand our perceptions. Now, I will like to ask you:

- What insights or information in this chapter caught you by surprise?
- Was there a particular fact or perspective that shifted your understanding of obesity?
- Reflecting on what you've learned, how might this influence your approach to health and lifestyle decisions moving forward?

I encourage you to engage in a meaningful conversation with someone close to you about a key takeaway from this chapter. Exploring how this newfound understanding could impact both of your health choices, deepens your connection and contributes to a ripple effect of wellness and awareness in your circles.

Chapter 2: The Power of Lifestyle Medicine

"Lifestyle Medicine is the art and science of helping individuals discover the healing power of their own lives. It's about choosing health with every decision we make."

Principles and Practices

Imagine lifestyle medicine as a journey to wellness, where every step you take is a choice towards better health. It's a transformative approach that transcends traditional medicine by focusing on how daily habits and routines can prevent, treat, and even reverse disease. Lifestyle medicine is grounded in six core principles:

Nutrition:
This is about more than just eating healthy; it's about nourishing your body. A diet rich in fruits, vegetables, whole grains, and lean proteins provides the essential nutrients your body needs to function optimally. For example, fiber-rich foods not only aid digestion but also help regulate blood sugar levels, reducing the risk of diabetes. Minimizing processed foods and sugars reduces the risk of chronic diseases like heart disease.

Physical Activity:
Regular exercise is a key component. This doesn't mean you need to run marathons; even a daily brisk walk can significantly improve cardiovascular health. Exercise helps control weight, strengthens the heart, and improves mental health by releasing endorphins, the body's natural mood lifters.

Stress Management:
In today's fast-paced world, managing stress is vital. Techniques like mindfulness, meditation, or even simple breathing exercises

can lower cortisol levels, reducing the risk of stress-related conditions like hypertension.

Adequate Sleep:
Quality sleep is as vital as diet and exercise. It's during sleep that your body repairs itself. Poor sleep can disrupt hormonal balance, leading to weight gain, irritability, and reduced cognitive function. Developing a sleep routine, like going to bed and waking up simultaneously every day, can significantly enhance sleep quality.

Avoiding Risky Substances:
This principle focuses on removing substances detrimental to health, like tobacco, and moderating alcohol consumption. Avoiding smoking reduces the risk of lung cancer and a multitude of respiratory conditions while limiting alcohol can prevent liver disease and help in weight management.

Healthy Relationships:
Positive social connections contribute to mental and emotional health. Being part of a supportive community can provide a sense of belonging and purpose, essential for mental well-being.

Lifestyle medicine is not just about tackling an existing condition; it's about overhauling your life to prioritize health in every aspect. It's a commitment to making choices that lead to a healthier, happier you. While we will explore these points in more depth in subsequent chapters, understanding these principles lays the foundation for the transformative power of lifestyle medicine.

Reflect on the Principles and Practices

So, you've just learned the core principles of lifestyle medicine, each serving as a stepping stone towards a healthier life.

- As you think about these principles, which one resonates with you the most right now, and why?
- Can you identify one small change you could make today that aligns with any of these principles?

Now, I want you to:

- Create a weekly chart and set a simple, achievable goal for each principle. Track your progress and note any changes in how you feel physically and mentally.

Science and Lifestyle: How Lifestyle Changes Impact Health

When science and lifestyle converge, we witness a profound impact on health. It's a synergy where evidence-based medical knowledge meets our daily choices, leading to transformative health outcomes.

1. The Science of Eating Right:
Let's consider nutrition first. Scientific studies consistently show the power of a balanced diet in preventing and managing diseases. For example, the Mediterranean diet, rich in fruits, vegetables, and healthy fats, has been linked to a lower risk of heart disease and stroke. It's not just about eating less; it's about eating right. Nutrient-dense foods provide the building blocks your body needs to repair itself, fight inflammation, and boost immunity.

2. The Power of Movement:
Exercise is another area where science and lifestyle intertwine. Regular physical activity reduces the risk of chronic diseases like diabetes, heart disease, and certain cancers. It's about finding an activity you enjoy and making it a part of your routine. The key is consistency, whether it's a dance class, a daily jog, or yoga. Exercise benefits not just the body but also the mind, helping to alleviate symptoms of depression and anxiety.

3. Stress Reduction and Health:
The impact of stress management on health is significant. Chronic stress can lead to a range of health issues, from hypertension to mental health disorders. Techniques like mindfulness and meditation aren't just relaxation practices; they're tools backed by science to lower stress hormones and promote well-being.

4. Sleep's Role in Wellness:
The importance of sleep can't be overstated. Research shows that adequate sleep is crucial for everything from maintaining a healthy weight to cognitive function. Poor sleep habits have been linked to a higher risk of obesity, diabetes, and even heart disease. You're taking a vital step in your health journey by improving your sleep hygiene – like establishing a regular sleep schedule and creating a restful environment.

5. The Impact of Substance Moderation:
The avoidance or moderation of harmful substances like tobacco and excessive alcohol has clear health benefits. For instance, quitting smoking can dramatically reduce the risk of lung cancer and improve respiratory health. Moderating alcohol intake can protect against liver disease and contribute to overall health.

6. Social Health as a Pillar:
Finally, the role of healthy relationships and social connections in overall well-being is increasingly recognized. A strong social network can lead to better mental health, lower stress levels, and even longer life expectancy.

In every aspect, lifestyle choices backed by scientific understanding can lead to significant health improvements. This chapter is about connecting those dots – understanding how the choices you make every day, based on solid scientific evidence, can lead to a healthier, more vibrant life.

Reflective Prompts:

- Have you experienced the benefits of any of these scientific principles in your own life?
- Which area (nutrition, physical activity, stress management, etc.) do you feel could use more attention in your life?

Now, let's create a simple exercise for you:

Choose one scientific insight that intrigued you. Plan a 30-day challenge to integrate this insight into your life. Journal the changes you observe.

The Holistic Approach: Combining Diet, Exercise, and Mindset

The essence of lifestyle medicine lies in its holistic approach. It's about integrating diet, exercise, and mindset into a unified strategy for health and well-being. This approach acknowledges that our health is not just a sum of isolated factors but a harmonious interplay of our physical, mental, and emotional selves.

1. Diet: More than Just Food Choices:
A holistic diet approach is not about strict dietary restrictions; it's about understanding and respecting your body's nutritional needs. It's recognizing that what you eat not only affects your waistline but also your energy levels, mood, and overall health. A balanced diet rich in whole foods provides essential nutrients that support bodily functions, improve immunity, and enhance mental clarity.

2. Exercise: Beyond Physical Fitness:
Exercise in a holistic sense is about more than just physical fitness; it's about finding joy and satisfaction in movement. It's about understanding how regular physical activity can strengthen your body, clear your mind, and elevate your mood. Whether it's a brisk walk in the park, a yoga session, or a dance class, exercise should be something that you look forward to, a celebration of what your body can do.

3. Mindset - The Power of Positive Thinking:
The role of mindset in health cannot be overstated. A positive mindset can be a powerful tool in managing stress, overcoming challenges, and maintaining motivation. It's about cultivating an attitude of gratitude, resilience, and self-compassion. This mental shift can influence every choice you make, from what you eat to how you respond to stress, and can significantly impact your overall health journey.

The beauty of the holistic approach is that it creates a positive feedback loop. Good nutrition boosts your energy for exercise; exercise improves your mood and mental clarity, and a positive mindset helps you make healthier food choices. Each element supports and enhances the others, leading to a healthier, more balanced you.

Chapter Thoughts:

We've explored the power of lifestyle medicine together, discovering how our everyday decisions significantly affect our health.

- Did any piece of these information transform the way you think about your health and daily habits?
- How might you apply a holistic approach to your lifestyle moving forward?

"Empower others through shared knowledge. Together, we can craft a healthier world."

Share an insight from this chapter with someone. Discussing these ideas can inspire change and foster a supportive community around health and wellness.

By engaging with these reflections and exercises, you're not just passively absorbing information; you're actively participating in your health journey. Every step, no matter how small, is a victory in the art of choosing health. Let's continue this journey with intention, compassion, and curiosity.

Chapter 3: Nutrition and Obesity

"Your diet is a bank account. Good food choices are good investments." – Bethenny Frankel.

The relationship between our diet and obesity is more than just a matter of calories in versus calories out. It's a complex interplay that significantly impacts our health and well-being.

Obesity typically develops when we consistently consume more calories than our body's burn. These extra calories, especially from foods high in fat and sugar, are stored as body fat. However, the story doesn't end with calorie counting. The type of food we eat is just as important as the quantity.

Consider the difference in nutritional value between 200 calories worth of a candy bar and 200 calories of fruit. The candy bar, laden with sugar and fat, might cause a quick spike in blood sugar and, soon after, a crash that leaves you hungry. The fruit, with its fiber and essential nutrients, offers a more gradual release of energy and longer-lasting satiety.

This distinction is crucial because different types of foods influence our bodies in different ways. They can affect our metabolism, the hormones that regulate our appetite, and even our brain chemistry related to hunger and satisfaction. Thus, understanding how our diet influences obesity is vital to managing and preventing it effectively. It's not just about losing weight; it's about nurturing our bodies with the right foods to support overall health.

Macronutrients: Essential Energy Sources

Now, let's look at another essential aspect of managing obesity effectively: understanding the roles of macronutrients, micronutrients, and hydration in our diet. This knowledge is key to making informed decisions about our food choices, which in turn, has a significant impact on our body weight and overall health.

- **Carbohydrates: The Fuel for Our Body**

Complex Carbohydrates:
Found in whole grains, fruits, and vegetables, these carbs are like long-burning logs on a fire – they provide sustained energy and are packed with fiber, aiding digestion and keeping you full longer.

Simple Carbohydrates:
Often found in sugary snacks and drinks, these are like quick-burning paper; they give a rapid energy spike followed by a crash, leading to hunger and potential overeating.

- **Proteins: The Building Blocks**

Lean Proteins:
Sources such as meats, fish, beans, and tofu not only repair and build body tissues but also play a crucial role in weight management. They help you feel full for longer, reducing the tendency to snack on unhealthy options.

Balanced Intake:
Including a source of protein in each meal can keep your energy levels steady throughout the day and support muscle health, which is especially important if you're incorporating exercise into your routine.

- **Fats: The Necessary Nutrient**

Healthy Fats are vital for brain health, hormone production, and overall cell function. Sources like avocados, nuts, and olive oil provide these essential fats without the adverse effects associated with saturated and trans fats found in many fried and processed foods.

Moderation and Choice:
The key is in the balance – ensuring that your intake of fats is mostly from healthy sources and in moderation.

Micronutrients: Vitamins and Minerals for Optimal Health

Vitamins A, D, E, and K: Supporting Diverse Bodily Functions

Vitamin A:
Essential for good vision and immune function, found in carrots, sweet potatoes, and leafy greens.

Vitamin D:
Crucial for bone health and immune response, obtained from exposure to sunlight, dairy products, and certain fish.

Vitamin E:
 An antioxidant that protects cells from damage, present in nuts, seeds, and vegetable oils.

Vitamin K:
Key in blood clotting and bone metabolism, found in green leafy vegetables and certain vegetable oils.

Minerals: Supporting Structural and Functional Needs

Calcium for Bones:

Essential for strong bones and teeth, dairy products and fortified plant milks are good sources.

Iron for Blood Health:
Found in meats and some beans, iron is crucial for carrying oxygen in the blood.

Potassium for Muscle Function:
Bananas and potatoes are great sources of potassium, helping with muscle function and cardiovascular health.

Hydration: More than Just Quenching Thirst

Water plays a critical role in our overall health. It's essential for digestion, nutrient transport, and regulating body temperature. The standard advice is to drink 8-10 cups of water daily, but this can vary based on individual activity levels, climate, and physical needs. Hydration isn't just about water; it also includes other fluids and hydrating foods like fruits and vegetables. Proper hydration aids in metabolism and helps maintain energy levels throughout the day.

Now, let's take a moment to reflect and engage more deeply with the concepts introduced thus far:

- ***Nutritional Choices and their Impact:***

Reflect on a day's worth of meals. Can you identify if your choices leaned more towards complex carbohydrates or simple ones? How might these choices be influencing your overall energy levels and feelings of satiety?

- ***Proteins in Your Diet:***

Think about the protein sources in your recent meals. Were they mostly lean and plant-based, or did you find yourself opting for options higher in saturated fats? How do you think these choices contribute to your feeling full and satisfied?

Fats: The Good vs. the Bad:

Assess your intake of fats over the past week. How often did you incorporate healthy fats into your diet, and in what forms? Can you spot any patterns of consuming saturated or Trans fats that you might want to change?

Exercises for You

1. *Carb Comparison Challenge:*

- For one day, try to replace simple carbohydrates with complex ones in your meals. Note any differences in how you feel, both in terms of energy levels and hunger, at the end of the day.

2. *Protein Power:*

- Experiment with adding a lean protein source to each meal for two days. Observe any changes in how long you feel full after eating and your overall energy levels.

3. *Healthy Fats Swap:*

- Identify one meal a day where you can switch out a saturated or trans-fat source for a healthy fat (think avocado instead of butter). Do this for a week and reflect on any changes in your mood, satiety, and overall health.

Mindful Eating: The Art of Being Present

- ***Understanding Mindful Eating:***

The Essence:
Mindful eating isn't just a diet strategy; it's a shift in how we perceive and interact with food. It's about engaging fully in your experience while eating – noticing your food's colors, smells, textures, and flavors and bringing a sense of awareness to every bite.

The Process:
Start by eating without distractions. Turn off the TV and put away your phone. Focus solely on your meal. Chew slowly, savoring each mouthful, and listen to your body's signals. Are you truly hungry or reaching for a second serving out of habit or emotion?

The Benefits:
This approach can transform eating from a mindless act to a deliberate and enjoyable experience. It helps regulate portion sizes naturally and can be an effective tool in weight management. Mindful eating also encourages a healthier relationship with food, fostering appreciation and enjoyment rather than guilt and restriction.

The Key Benefits

- Preventing Overeating: Eating slowly and mindfully gives your body time to recognize when it's full, reducing the likelihood of overeating.

- Addressing Emotional Eating: Mindful eating helps you recognize emotional triggers that lead to unnecessary snacking or overindulgence. It shifts the focus from eating for comfort to eating for nourishment.

Portion Control: Balancing Food Intake

<u>Importance of Portion Control:</u>

- Portion control is essential for managing caloric intake. Eating portions that are too large, even of healthy foods, can contribute to weight gain.

- It also ensures you're getting a balanced intake of nutrients. By controlling portion sizes, you can include a variety of foods in your diet without overindulging in any one type.

<u>Practical Tips for Portion Control:</u>

- ***Visual Cues:*** Use your hand as a guide – a fist for vegetables, a palm for protein, and a cupped hand for carbs.

- ***Plate Method:*** Try using smaller plates to reduce portion sizes naturally. This tricks the mind into feeling satisfied with less food.

- ***Mindful Serving:*** Serve food on your plate instead of eating straight from the package. This allows you to be conscious of the amount you're consuming.

<u>Synergistic Effect</u>

- Mindful eating and portion control complement each other. While mindful eating helps you tune into your body's hunger and fullness cues, portion control provides a practical framework for managing the quantity of food you consume.

- Cultivating Healthy Habits: Together, they form a holistic approach to eating that can lead to long-term changes in dietary behavior and weight management. It's not about restrictive dieting; it's about creating a sustainable, balanced relationship with food.

Reflections:

1. **A Moment of Mindfulness:**

   - Reflect on your last meal. Were you fully present, or were your thoughts elsewhere? Consider how being more mindful could change your eating experience.

2. **Portion Perception:**

   - Think about a time you ate more than you intended. How did portion control (or the lack of it) play a role? What visual cues could have helped you eat just enough?

Exercises for You:

1. **Mindful Meal Challenge:**

   - For your next meal, commit to eating without distractions. No TV, no phone—just you and your meal. Focus on the taste, texture, and aroma of your food. Chew slowly and assess your hunger after each bite. How does this change your eating experience?

2. **Portion Control Practice:**

    - Use the hand guide for your next meal to measure portions without a scale. A fist for vegetables, a palm for proteins, and a cupped hand for carbs. Notice any differences in how satisfied you feel afterwards.

3. **Mindful Snacking:**

    - Next time you reach for a snack, pause. Are you truly hungry, or is it boredom or emotion driving you? If you decide to snack, do so mindfully, savoring each bite and stopping when you're satisfied.

Creating a Healthy Eating Environment

Setting the Scene for Mindful Eating:

- *Environment Matters*: The atmosphere in which you eat can significantly impact how you eat. To encourage mindful eating, create a calm and pleasant dining environment. This might mean eating at a well-set table, free from the distractions of electronic devices or stressful conversations. It's about making mealtime a peaceful, dedicated moment for nourishment.

- *Engaging the Senses:* Enhance your dining area with elements that please the senses – perhaps some gentle background music, comfortable seating, or visually appealing dinnerware. This sensory engagement can enrich the eating experience, making it more satisfying and relaxing.

Eating Without Distractions:

- *Mindful Presence:* Encourage eating without distractions. This means turning off the TV, putting away phones, and avoiding eating while working or driving. By focusing solely on your meal, you can better tune into your body's hunger and fullness cues and enjoy each bite more fully.

- *Family Meals:* If possible, make mealtimes a family affair. Eating with others can provide a sense of connection and shared enjoyment. It's also an opportunity to model healthy eating habits for children, teaching them the importance of a balanced diet and a mindful approach to food.

Cultivating Mindful Habits around Food:

- *Pausing before Eating:* Take a moment before you start eating to appreciate the meal in front of you. This pause can help center your thoughts and transition your focus to the act of eating.

- *Appreciating Your Food:* Acknowledge the effort that went into preparing your meal, whether you cooked it, someone else, or even prepared in a restaurant. This gratitude can deepen your connection to the food and enhance the overall experience.

Balancing Mindfulness and Practicality:

- While it's ideal to create a perfect eating environment for every meal, it's important to balance mindfulness with the practicalities of daily life. Even when you can't control your environment, you can still practice mindful eating by focusing on your food and listening to your body's signals.

- Creating a healthy eating environment isn't about perfection; it's about making small, mindful changes that add up over time. By cultivating these practices, you can transform your eating habits, leading to more enjoyable and healthful meal experiences.

Addressing Emotional Eating

Emotional eating, the act of consuming food in response to feelings rather than hunger, is a common challenge. It's an area where understanding and strategy can bring about significant positive changes in both eating habits and overall emotional health.

Difference between Emotional and Physical Hunger

Recognizing Emotional Hunger:
Emotional hunger often arises suddenly and demands instant satisfaction with specific comfort foods, usually high in sugar, fat, or both. It's like a sudden craving for a specific type of food rather than just food in general.

Distinguishing Physical Hunger:
In contrast, physical hunger develops gradually and can be satisfied with various foods. It's the body's natural response to needing energy and comes with signals like a growling stomach.

Mindful Response:
By tuning into these cues and asking yourself whether you're really hungry or just seeking to feed an emotion, you can break the emotional eating cycle.
Strategies for Managing Emotional Eating:

Find Alternate Coping Mechanisms:
When you feel the urge to eat in response to an emotion, pause to consider other activities that might provide comfort or distraction.

This could be anything from walking, engaging in a hobby, or calling a friend.

Emotional Awareness:
 Sometimes, simply acknowledging your emotions can diminish their power over your eating habits. Writing in a journal or talking to someone can help you process these feelings.

Reflections: So, we have explore the environment's role in mindful eating and the importance of eating without distractions, let's reflect on how we can integrate these concepts into our lives more actively.

Assess Your Eating Environment:

- Think about where you usually eat your meals. Is it conducive to mindful eating, or are there distractions that take away from the experience? How can you make your dining space more inviting and focused on the act of eating?

Emotional vs. Physical Hunger:

- Reflect on a recent instance where you might have eaten in response to emotions rather than actual hunger. How did you differentiate between emotional hunger and physical hunger, and what alternative coping mechanisms could you have used?

Exercises for you:

1. Creating a Mindful Eating Space:

For your next meal, make a conscious effort to create a calming and enjoyable dining environment. This could involve setting the table, playing some soft music, or even lighting a candle. Notice if this change impacts your eating experience.

2. Mindful Meal with Family or Friends:

Plan a meal where everyone commits to eating mindfully, without distractions. Discuss the experience afterwards. Did it change how you ate or how you felt during and after the meal?

3. Pause and Appreciate:

Before you begin eating, take a moment to look at your food and appreciate where it came from and the effort that went into preparing it. Try to carry this sense of gratitude and presence throughout the meal.

4. Identify Emotional Hunger:

Next time you feel a sudden urge to eat, pause and reflect on what you're feeling. Are you physically hungry, or are there emotions you might be trying to feed? Write down what you're feeling and consider other ways to address those emotions.

Meal Planning: Simple and Nutritious Meal Ideas

Meal planning is a powerful tool in managing nutrition effectively. It involves thinking ahead and preparing meals that are both nutritious and enjoyable. This practice helps control portions and calorie intake and ensures a balanced intake of essential nutrients.

The Basics of Meal Planning

Start with a Template: Plan your meals around balanced nutrition. A good rule of thumb is to fill half your plate with fruits and vegetables, a quarter with lean protein, and a quarter with whole grains.

Variety is Key: Incorporate different foods each week to ensure a range of nutrients and keep meals interesting.

Practical Tips for Effective Meal Planning

Batch Cooking: Prepare and cook meals in bulk. This saves time and ensures you have healthy options readily available.

Use a Shopping List: Plan your grocery shopping based on your meal plan. Stick to your list to avoid impulse purchases.

Embrace Leftovers: Cook a little extra to prepare meals for the next day, reducing the temptation to opt for less healthy options.

Simple Meal Ideas

- Breakfast: Whole grain oats with berries, a scoop of Greek yogurt, an omelet with spinach and mushrooms.

- Lunch: Grilled chicken salad with various veggies; a quinoa and black bean bowl with avocado and salsa.

- <u>Dinner:</u> Baked salmon with roasted sweet potatoes and green beans; vegetable stir-fry with tofu and brown rice.

Snack Ideas

Healthy snacking is important, too. Opt for fruits, nuts, and carrot sticks with hummus, or yogurt with a handful of granola.

Stay Flexible and Listen to Your Body

While meal planning is about preparation, it's also important to remain flexible and listen to your body's hunger cues. Adjust portions and meal components as needed.

Making Meal Planning a Family Activity

Involve family members in the planning process. This makes it easier and helps inculcate healthy eating habits among all family members.

Meal planning doesn't have to be a chore. With a little creativity and preparation, it can be a rewarding process contributing significantly to your health journey. These guidelines simplify the process, making it more approachable and sustainable in the long term.

A Sample Week of Meal Planning

Here's a sample week-long plan to give you a clearer picture of how meal planning can work in practice. This plan balances nutritional needs with variety to keep meals interesting and healthy.

DAY	MEAL TIME	MENU
Day 1	Breakfast	Greek yogurt with mixed berries and a sprinkle of chia seeds.
	Lunch	Turkey and avocado wrap with whole grain tortilla, side of carrot sticks.
	Dinner	Grilled salmon with a quinoa and spinach salad.
Day 2	Breakfast	Scrambled eggs with sautéed kale and whole grain toast.
	Lunch	Lentil soup with a side of mixed greens salad.
	Dinner	Chicken stir-fry with assorted veggies and brown rice.
Day 3	Breakfast	Smoothie with banana, spinach, almond milk, and a scoop of protein powder.
	Lunch	Quinoa bowl with black beans, corn, diced tomatoes, and avocado.
	Dinner	Baked cod with roasted Brussels sprouts and sweet potatoes.
Day 4	Breakfast	Oatmeal topped with sliced almonds and apple slices.
	Lunch	Chickpea and vegetable salad with olive oil and lemon dressing.
	Dinner	Turkey meatballs with whole wheat spaghetti and marinara sauce.
Day 5	Breakfast	Whole grain toast with peanut butter

		and banana slices.
	Lunch	Tuna salad over mixed greens with cucumber and cherry tomatoes.
	Dinner	Vegetable curry with lentils served over brown rice.
Day 6	Breakfast	Cottage cheese with pineapple chunks and walnuts.
	Lunch	Whole grain pita stuffed with grilled veggies and hummus.
	Dinner	Beef and vegetable kebabs with a side of quinoa tabbouleh.
Day 7	Breakfast	Veggie omelet with a side of mixed fruit.
	Lunch	Leftover vegetable curry with a fresh green salad.
	Dinner	Baked chicken breast with asparagus and a side of wild rice.

Snacks (Choose 2-3 per day)

- A handful of almonds or walnuts.
- A piece of fruit (apple, orange, or a bunch of grapes).
- Carrot and celery sticks with hummus.
- Greek yogurt with a tablespoon of honey.
- A slice of cheese with whole grain crackers.

Hydration:
Aim to drink at least 8-10 glasses of water throughout the day. Herbal teas and infusions can also be included.

This meal plan is just a guide and can be adjusted based on personal preferences, dietary needs, and specific health goals. The idea is to use it as a template to build your own meal plans that fit your lifestyle and nutritional requirements.

So, you have learned a lot throughout this chapter. Now, let's take a moment to reflect on how you can incorporate the knowledge to enhance nutritional well-being and make mealtime an enjoyable part of our day.

Your Personal Meal Planning Experience:

- Reflect on your current meal planning habits. What challenges do you face in planning nutritious meals, and how can the tips provided help overcome those obstacles?

Variety in Diet:

- Consider the variety of foods in your typical weekly diet. Are there food groups you're neglecting? How can you incorporate more diversity to ensure a balanced intake of nutrients?

Exercises for you

Create Your Meal Plan:

- Using the template suggested (half fruits and vegetables, a quarter lean protein, a quarter whole grains), plan out your meals for the next three days. Aim for variety and balance. Share your plan with a family member or friend for accountability.

Batch Cooking Session:

- Schedule a batch cooking session to prepare multiple meals in advance. Notice if this helps reduce stress around meal times and how it impacts your food choices throughout the week.

Grocery Shopping Challenge:

- On your next grocery trip, stick strictly to your shopping list based on your meal plan. Reflect on how this strategy affects your purchases and if it helps you make healthier food choices.

Leftover Creativity:

- Take a meal you've cooked and figure out how to repurpose the leftovers into a new meal for the next day. For instance, turn last night's grilled chicken into a hearty salad for lunch. This exercise encourages creativity and reduces food waste.

Family Meal Planning:

- Involve your family in the meal planning process for a week. Discuss everyone's favorite meals and how they can be made healthier. This shared activity can lead to better adherence to the meal plan and foster healthier eating habits for all.

Cauliflower: A Versatile Substitute for Grains and Fufu Powder

In recent years, cauliflower has emerged as a superstar in the world of healthy eating, celebrated for its versatility and nutritional benefits. This humble vegetable has become a favored substitute for grains and traditional fufu powder, offering a low-carb alternative that aligns well with various dietary goals, especially for those focusing on weight loss and better health management.

Why Cauliflower?
Cauliflower stands out due to its remarkable ability to mimic the texture and flavor of starchy favorites when processed correctly. Rich in vitamins C, K, B6 and an excellent source of dietary fiber, cauliflower supports a healthy immune system, promotes digestion, and can contribute to lowering inflammation. Its low calorie and carbohydrate content makes it an ideal choice for individuals looking to reduce their carb intake without sacrificing satisfaction or flavor.

Cauliflower as Grain Substitute:
Transformed into "rice," cauliflower provides a fantastic alternative to traditional grains like white rice or couscous. Simply pulse cauliflower florets in a food processor until they reach a rice-like consistency, then lightly sauté or steam to perfection. This cauliflower rice can serve as the base for various dishes, from stir-fries to pilafs, seamlessly incorporated into meals for a nutritious boost.

Cauliflower in Fufu:
For those who enjoy fufu but are mindful of carb intake, cauliflower offers a compelling solution. Combining steamed and mashed cauliflower with a small amount of psyllium husk for binding can create a fufu-like consistency that's both satisfying and healthy. This cauliflower fufu pairs beautifully with traditional soups and stews, allowing you to enjoy your favorite dishes in a lighter, more nutritious manner.

Incorporating Cauliflower into Your Diet:

- **Start Small:** If you're new to cauliflower as a substitute, integrate it into one meal a week, gradually increasing as you become accustomed to the texture and flavor.

- **Get Creative:** Explore different recipes and cooking methods. Cauliflower's mild taste makes it a blank canvas for various flavors and seasonings.

- **Mix It Up:** Combine cauliflower with other vegetables or grains to diversify your nutrient intake while enjoying its benefits.

Embracing cauliflower as a substitute for grains and fufu powder is more than just a dietary change; it's a step towards a healthier, more balanced lifestyle. With its nutritional profile and versatility, cauliflower allows you to enjoy your favorite meals in a way that supports your health and wellness goals.

Chapter 4: Integrating Mediterranean Diet, Intermittent Fasting, Keto and DASH Diet for Weight loss

"The secret to weight loss is not to eat less, but to eat right. The Mediterranean diet, Intermittent Fasting, and DASH Diet illuminate the path to health through wisdom in eating."

I n the earlier section, we've explored how diet is essential in managing weight and enhancing overall health. But have you considered how specific diets, tailored to unique lifestyles and health goals, can be even more impactful? Let's look into the Mediterranean diet, Intermittent Fasting, and the DASH Diet, each offering its blueprint for nurturing your body and supporting weight loss.

The Mediterranean Diet – a taste of longevity

- The Mediterranean diet is celebrated for its delicious flavors and numerous health benefits. It's centered around plant-based foods, lean proteins, and healthy fats, particularly olive oil, rich in monounsaturated fats.

- This diet encourages consuming fish and poultry at least twice a week, enjoying meals with family and friends, and even allowing for a glass of red wine, making it a diet and a lifestyle. Whole grains, nuts, and seeds provide fiber and nutrients, while fruits and vegetables offer a variety of vitamins and antioxidants, supporting everything from brain to heart health.

- The Mediterranean diet's emphasis on whole foods and natural ingredients contributes to sustainable weight loss and a reduced risk of chronic diseases.

Intermittent Fasting – timing is everything

- Intermittent Fasting (IF) challenges the traditional three-meals-a-day routine by introducing periods of fasting and eating. It's not just about what you eat but when you eat, creating windows where your body taps into fat stores for energy.

- This process not only aids in weight loss but also improves insulin sensitivity, reduces inflammation, and may enhance longevity. Whether you choose the 16/8 method, alternate-day fasting, or the 5:2 approach, IF promotes metabolic flexibility and encourages a mindful relationship with food. It's adaptable to your lifestyle, making it a practical choice for many looking to lose weight or improve their metabolic health.

The DASH Diet (Dietary Approaches to Stop Hypertension)

- Originally developed to lower blood pressure, the DASH Diet also offers a balanced approach to weight loss. It focuses on nutrient-rich foods that reduce sodium intake and increase potassium, calcium, and magnesium—key nutrients that help lower blood pressure.

- By emphasizing fruits, vegetables, whole grains, and lean proteins, the DASH Diet supports heart health and encourages a reduction in the consumption of red meat, salt, added sugars, and fat. It's a structured plan that helps you shed pounds and cultivate eating habits that are good for your heart and overall health.

The Keto Diet

- The Keto Diet is a high-fat, moderate protein and low-carbohydrate diet designed to put your body into a state of ketosis, where it burns fat for fuel instead of carbohydrates. This shift can lead to significant weight loss and may have benefits for certain medical conditions.

- This diet plan dramatically reduces carb intake, replacing it with healthy fats and moderate protein levels. Staples of the Keto Diet include meats, fatty fish, eggs, butter, cheese, nuts, avocados, low-carb vegetables, and oils like coconut or olive oil. By limiting carbs to 20-50 grams per day, the body is forced to use alternative fuel sources.

- The Keto Diet's emphasis on fats over carbs can potentially lead to improvements in blood sugar levels, cholesterol, and triglycerides, contributing to better heart health. However, because of its restrictive nature, it may not be suitable for everyone, and it's important to consult with a healthcare professional before starting, especially for individuals with pre-existing health conditions.

Staying Hydrated – more than just water

- Hydration is essential across all diets. It aids in digestion, helps regulate body temperature, and supports metabolic processes. To keep hydrated, aim for at least 64 ounces of fluid daily, utilizing tools like time-marked water bottles to track your intake. Enhancing water with fruits, coconut milk, or electrolyte granules makes it more enjoyable and supports your body's hydration needs. Remember, a well-hydrated body functions better, aiding in weight loss and overall health.

Seeking Professional Guidance:

Embarking on a new diet can be a transformative journey best navigated with professional support. A registered dietitian can provide personalized advice, ensuring your diet aligns with your health requirements and lifestyle. Sustainable weight management is about making informed lifestyle changes, not temporary fixes. A professional can guide you through this process, helping you to achieve lasting results.

- In considering these diets, reflect on your personal health goals, lifestyle, and preferences. Whether it's the rich flavors of the Mediterranean, the strategic eating windows of Intermittent Fasting, or the balanced approach of the DASH Diet, there's a path for everyone. With hydration as your constant companion and professional guidance to lead the way, you're set on a course for healthier living and sustainable weight loss.

What can you do today?

- Reflect on your current lifestyle and eating habits. Which of these diets resonates most with you in terms of preferences, feasibility, and goals? Why?

<u>Exercises for you</u>

1. Mediterranean Diet Meal Planning:

Plan a day's meals inspired by the Mediterranean diet. Include a variety of plant-based foods, whole grains, and a source of healthy fat like olive oil. Share your plan with a friend or family member and discuss the potential health benefits.

2. Intermittent Fasting Trial:

Choose one form of Intermittent Fasting to try for a week. Keep a journal of your experience, noting how you feel physically and mentally. Reflect on how this eating pattern might fit into your long-term health goals.

3. DASH Diet Grocery Challenge:

Next time you go grocery shopping, try to adhere to the DASH diet's guidelines. Focus on purchasing fruits, vegetables, whole grains, and lean proteins, and limit high-sodium and sugary foods. Notice any changes in your shopping habits or meal choices.

4. Hydration Habit Tracking:

For one week, monitor your fluid intake, aiming for at least 64 ounces a day. Experiment with adding fruits or coconut milk to enhance flavor. Reflect on how staying well-hydrated affects your energy levels, appetite, and overall well-being.

Tip for Connection:

"Food is more than just nutrition—it's a gateway to a healthier life and connection."

Host a dinner where you prepare a meal based on one of the diets discussed. Invite friends or family to experience the flavors and discuss the health benefits. This not only enriches your understanding but also spreads awareness and encourages a community around healthy eating.

Chapter 5: Physical Activity and Weight Loss

"Exercise should be regarded as a tribute to the heart." – Gene Tunney.

The connection between exercise and weight management is profound, impacting much more than just the number on the scale. Let's break down this relationship and understand why exercise is crucial in weight loss and overall health.

1. Calorie Burning: The Basic Equation
At its simplest, weight loss is about burning more calories than you consume. Exercise, in this context, is your powerhouse. It's like having extra gear in a car – it helps you reach your weight loss goals faster. Whether it's a brisk walk, a spin class, or lifting weights, each activity increases your calorie burn, contributing to the calorie deficit needed for weight loss.

2. Metabolic Boost: Keeping the Engine Running
Regular physical activity doesn't just burn calories while you're doing it but also increases your metabolism, meaning you burn more calories even at rest. It's like upgrading your car's engine for better fuel efficiency. This metabolic boost is significant as you lose weight and your body naturally burns fewer calories.

3. Muscle Matters: Beyond the Calorie Burn
While aerobic exercises are great for burning calories, strength training is crucial for building muscle. Muscle tissue burns more calories than fat tissue, even when you're not moving. Think of muscle as an investment in a calorie-burning bank account – the more you have, the higher your daily calorie expenditure, even when you're just sitting around.

4. The Ripple Effect: Beyond Weight Loss
The benefits of exercise extend far beyond weight loss. It improves cardiovascular health, increases endurance, and reduces the risk of chronic diseases like diabetes and heart disease. Additionally, regular physical activity improves mental health, reducing symptoms of depression and anxiety. It's a ripple effect; you start exercising for weight loss but gain much more overall health and well-being.

5. Hormonal Harmony: Exercise and Appetite Regulation
Regular exercise can also help regulate hormones that control appetite. For instance, it can decrease levels of ghrelin, the hunger hormone, and increase leptin levels, which signals fullness to the brain. This hormonal balance can help curb overeating, making it easier to stick to a healthy diet and promote weight loss.

6. Psychological Benefits: A Sense of Achievement
Finally, the psychological aspect of regularly exercising cannot be overstated. Each time you complete a workout, you build physical strength and mental resilience. This sense of accomplishment, the 'I can do this' feeling, is pivotal. It builds confidence and commitment, essential for long-term weight management and overall health.

Finding Your Fit: Tailoring Physical Activity to Individual Needs

Your exercise regime must be customized to your needs, preferences, and lifestyle. This personalization is key to making physical activity both effective and sustainable.

1. Assessing Personal Preferences and Lifestyle:
Start by reflecting on what you enjoy. Do you prefer the solitude and focus of weightlifting, the social aspect of group classes, or the serenity of yoga? Your exercise choices should resonate with your personality. It's like choosing a favorite flavor of ice cream – the right choice makes the experience much more enjoyable.

Consider your daily routine. If you're a morning person, capitalize on that energy with an AM workout. Night owls might prefer an evening jog. Fitting exercise into your natural rhythm increases the likelihood of sticking with it.

2. Understanding Your Body's Needs:
Be mindful of any physical limitations or health conditions. If you have joint pain, swimming or cycling might be more comfortable than running. The key is to work with your body, not against it.

Factor in your current fitness level. Starting with overly ambitious workouts can lead to discouragement or injury. Begin at a comfortable level and gradually ramp up the intensity.

3. Setting Realistic and Enjoyable Goals:
Goals should be challenging yet achievable. If this is your first time running, don't start with a marathon. Begin with shorter distances and progressively increase your goal.
Incorporate activities you genuinely enjoy. If dance makes you happy, a Zumba class might appeal more than a treadmill. Enjoyment is a powerful motivator in maintaining regular exercise.

4. Variety for Sustained Engagement:

A mix of different types of exercise can prevent boredom and work different muscle groups. Combine cardio exercises like running or cycling with strength training and flexibility exercises like yoga or Pilates.

Changing up your routine also prevents fitness plateaus. Your body gets used to a specific type of exercise over time, so variety keeps challenging it.

5. Social Support and Accountability:
Working out with friends, joining a fitness class, or even participating in online fitness communities can provide motivation and accountability. It's like having a workout family; they can cheer you on and keep you on track.

Personal trainers or fitness coaches can also provide personalized guidance and help tailor your fitness plan to your goals.

6. Listening to Your Body and Adjusting Accordingly:
Pay attention to how your body responds to different activities. If something feels wrong, modify your approach.

Regularly reassess your routine. As you get fitter, your needs and capacities will change. Your exercise plan should evolve with you.

Finding the right fit for your physical activity is a journey of exploration and self-discovery. It's about creating a workout routine that feels less like a chore and more like a rewarding part of your day – something you look forward to, not something you must endure.

About Your Exercise Journey:

- Consider your current level of physical activity. What forms of exercise do you enjoy, and how can you incorporate more of them into your weekly routine?
- Think about any barriers that have kept you from being more active. How can you overcome these obstacles to make exercise a regular part of your life?

Action Plan:

Create a Weekly Exercise Schedule: Draft a plan that incorporates different types of activities you enjoy. Aim for a mix that includes cardiovascular exercises, strength training, and flexibility workouts. Share this plan with a friend or family member to help keep you accountable.

Discover What You Love: Experiment with at least two new types of physical activities this week. Try something outside your comfort zone, whether it's a dance class, a yoga session, or a new hiking trail. Note how you feel during and after each activity.

Motivational Tips

Set Achievable Goals: Write down three realistic fitness goals for the next month. Ensure they are specific, measurable, and attainable. Revisit these goals weekly to track your progress.

Celebrate Small Wins: Identify small milestones within your fitness journey, such as completing a workout without stopping, reaching a new personal best, or simply sticking to your exercise schedule for the week. Celebrate these achievements in a way that feels rewarding to you.

Social Support and Engagement:

Buddy Up: Partner with a friend or family member who has similar fitness goals. Plan regular workout sessions together, whether in person or virtually. This not only makes exercising more fun but also adds a layer of accountability.

Join a Community: Explore local or online fitness communities where you can share experiences, challenges, and successes.

Engaging with like-minded individuals can provide additional motivation and support.

Thoughts:

- After integrating these exercises and reflections into your routine, reflect on any changes you've noticed in your approach to physical activity. Has your motivation increased? Do you find yourself looking forward to your workouts more?
- How have the psychological benefits of exercise, such as improved mood and resilience, impacted other areas of your life?

Share your experiences with a friend, what's worked for you, and any tips that have helped you along the way. Your story could be the encouragement they need to take the first step towards a healthier lifestyle.

Overcoming Barriers – Time Management and Motivation

Navigating the obstacles of time management and motivation in exercise is akin to solving a complex puzzle. It requires strategy, patience, and a bit of creativity. Let's explore ways to overcome these common barriers and make physical activity a consistent part of your life.

1. Time Management: Making Room for Exercise

Finding Time: Look at your schedule and identify pockets of time dedicated to exercise. It might be waking up 30 minutes earlier, using lunch breaks for a quick walk, or scheduling a workout session like an important meeting.

Prioritize Exercise: Recognize physical activity as a non-negotiable part of your routine, like eating or sleeping. It's not about finding time; it's about making time.

Plan Ahead: Lay out your workout clothes the night before or pack your gym bag in advance. These small acts of preparation reduce friction and make it easier to stick to your plan.

2. Motivation: Fueling Your Exercise Journey

Set Clear, Attainable Goals: Motivation thrives on achievement. Set small, realistic goals and celebrate when you reach them. It's like climbing a staircase – reaching each step gives you the boost to take the next one.

Find Your 'Why': Identify personal reasons for exercising. It could be to improve health, feel better, or keep up with your kids. This personal connection can be a powerful motivator.

Track Progress: Use a journal, an app, or a fitness tracker to monitor your progress. Seeing improvements in distance, speed, or endurance can be incredibly motivating.

3. Overcoming Psychological Barriers:

Combat Negative Thoughts: Replace thoughts like "I can't do this" with "I'm doing this step by step." Positive self-talk can be a significant game-changer.

Visualize Success: Imagine the satisfaction of achieving your goals. Visualization can be a potent tool in maintaining focus and motivation.

4. Building a Support System:

Seek Support from Friends and Family: Share your fitness goals with loved ones. They can offer encouragement, join you in workouts, or hold you accountable.

Join a Community: Whether it's a local running club, a yoga class, or an online fitness community, being part of a group provides a sense of belonging and motivation.

5. Making Exercise Enjoyable:

Choose Activities You Love: Exercise shouldn't be a punishment. Try cycling, swimming, or a dance class if you dread the treadmill. When you enjoy the activity, it doesn't feel like a chore.

Mix It Up: Keep things interesting by varying your workouts. Routine can lead to boredom, so try new activities or change your workout environment.

Remember, the journey to regular physical activity is unique for each person. It's about finding what works for you, overcoming hurdles, and embracing exercise as an integral part of your life. With the right strategies, you can turn time management and motivation challenges into stepping stones for success.

A Comprehensive 1-Week Exercise Routine: Fun and Enjoyable!

Creating a week-long exercise routine that's both effective and enjoyable is like planning a mini-adventure. Each day brings something different, keeping things fresh and exciting. Here's a detailed, one-week plan that balances various types of exercise to cater to different fitness levels and interests.

- **Day 1: Cardio Kickstart**

Morning:
Start your week with an energizing 30-minute walk or jog. Whether it's around your neighborhood or at a local park, the goal is to get your heart rate up and muscles warmed.

Evening:
Wind down with 15 minutes of stretching or yoga to keep your muscles supple and flexible.

- **Day 2: Strength Training Focus**

Morning or Afternoon:
Dedicate about 30-40 minutes to strength training. This can include bodyweight exercises like push-ups, squats, and lunges or using weights if you have them. Remember to target different muscle groups.

Tip: If you're new to strength training, follow an online tutorial to ensure proper form.

- **Day 3: Fun Activity Day**

Choose an Activity You Love:
Dedicate this day to doing a physical activity you enjoy. It could be a dance class, a round of golf, or even a vigorous gardening session. Aim for at least 30 minutes of continuous activity.

- **Day 4: Midweek Stretch and Stabilize**

Yoga or Pilates:
Engage in a yoga or Pilate's session to stretch out your muscles and improve core stability. Plenty of online classes are available that cater to all levels, lasting anywhere from 20 minutes to an hour.

- **Day 5: High-Intensity Interval Training (HIIT)**

Morning or Evening:
Inject some intensity with a HIIT session. This could be a circuit of exercises performed at high intensity for short bursts (like 30 seconds), followed by brief rest periods.

Tip: You can find many HIIT workouts online that require no equipment and can be done in a small space.

- **Day 6: Active Recovery**

Light Activity:
Engage in a light, active recovery day. This might mean a leisurely bike ride, a gentle swim, or a brisk walk. The idea is to move your body without straining it.

- **Day 7: Adventure or Leisure Day**

Choose an Outdoor Activity:
Depending on your interests, go for a hike, a long bike ride, or perhaps a kayaking session if you're near water. If you prefer something more leisurely, a long walk in a scenic area or park can be a great way to end the week.

- *Daily:*

Morning and/or Evening:

Incorporate at least 10-15 minutes of stretching or light yoga to keep your body flexible and prevent stiffness.

<u>Notes:</u>
Customization: Feel free to swap days around to fit your schedule or replace activities with those you enjoy more.

<u>*Hydration:*</u>
Stay hydrated throughout the week, especially during intense workouts.
Listen to Your Body: If you feel fatigued or sore, allow yourself a lighter workout or extra rest day.

- This routine is designed to be a guide and inspiration. It combines various types of exercise to keep things interesting and enjoyable while ensuring a balanced approach to fitness. Let it be a starting point for crafting a routine that excites and motivates you.

Chapter 6: Behavior Change for Lasting Results

"Changing behavior is like changing tires on a moving car. Challenging, but not impossible if you've got the right tools and a bit of a daredevil streak."

Eating is more than just a physical act of nourishment; it's often intertwined with emotions and psychology. Understanding this can be like trying to solve a mystery where your feelings are the clues.

1. Emotional Triggers:

Emotional triggers are those moments when you find yourself halfway through a tub of ice cream without knowing how you got there. These triggers might be stress, boredom, sadness, or even joy. Recognizing these emotional cues is the first step toward managing them. It's about learning to differentiate between hunger that comes from the stomach and 'hunger' that comes from the heart or mind.

Sometimes, we eat not because our body needs it but because our emotions demand it. This awareness is crucial. It's like being a detective in your own life, observing and understanding why you reach for certain foods at certain times. It's not just about controlling what you eat but understanding why you eat.

2. Mindful Eating:

This is like putting your brain in the driver's seat before you eat. It involves paying attention to your food, savoring each bite, and knowing your hunger and fullness cues. Imagine treating every meal like a first date – you'd pay attention, savor the moment, and probably wouldn't show up in sweatpants. Mindful eating is about creating a connection with your food that transcends the physical act of eating where you engage all your senses – noticing the aroma, the texture, the taste, and even the sound of your food.

This practice encourages a deeper appreciation of your meals, turning each eating experience into a moment of mindfulness and reflection. By eating mindfully, you become more in tune with your body's true needs, helping to prevent overeating and making mealtime a more satisfying, nourishing experience

Building Healthy Habits: Steps for Lasting Lifestyle Changes

Creating lasting healthy habits is like teaching an old dog new tricks; it might take a bit of time and patience, but it's definitely possible and quite rewarding.

Start Small and Simple:

- Begin with manageable changes. If your salad days are far behind you, don't leap into a diet of only greens.

- Start by introducing one vegetable to your dinner plate.

- Think of it like dipping your toes in the pool before diving in.

- It's about easing into new habits, not shocking your system. For example, if you're not used to exercising, start with a daily 10-minute walk rather than an intense hour at the gym. Small steps are less daunting and more likely to become permanent fixtures in your routine.

Consistency is Key:
Stick with your new habit until it feels less like a chore and more like a part of your routine. It's like wearing a new hat: awkward at first, but soon you can't leave the house without it. The key here is regularity. If you're trying to drink more water, set reminders at intervals throughout the day. Over time, these small actions become ingrained, and before you know it, they're part of your everyday life, as natural as brushing your teeth.

Build on Success:
 Once a small change becomes part of your daily life, add another one. If you've successfully cut down on soda, next, work on reducing sugar in your coffee. It's like building a tower; make sure the base is strong before adding more layers. Celebrate each victory, no matter how small. These successes are the bricks of your building, each strengthening your resolve and proving to yourself that you can make these changes.

Celebrate Small Wins:
 Got through a week without binge eating? Pat yourself on the back or treat yourself to a movie. Celebrating small victories gives you the motivation to keep going. Acknowledge every step forward. This reinforcement can be a powerful tool in maintaining momentum. Think of it as giving yourself a gold star for each achievement. These celebrations make the journey enjoyable and rewarding.

Make it Fun:
If exercise feels like a punishment, find an activity you enjoy. Hate running? Maybe you'll like swimming or dancing. The key is to make it enjoyable so it doesn't feel like a punishment. Create a playlist of your favorite songs for your workout, or find a scenic route for your walks. When you associate these new habits with pleasure and enjoyment, you're more likely to stick with them.

Find a Buddy:
Sometimes, the journey is easier with company. Pair up with a friend who has similar health goals. It's like having a partner in a three-legged race – you keep each other balanced and moving forward. This companionship can motivate and make the process feel less like work and more like socializing.

Be Patient and Kind to Yourself:
 Change takes time, and slip-ups will happen. Instead of beating yourself up, acknowledge the hiccup and get back on track. It's about progress, not perfection. Remember, every journey faces bumps in the road, and that's okay. Be as compassionate to yourself as you would be to a friend in the same situation.

Remember, building healthy habits is a journey. There's no express train; it's more like a scenic route with plenty of stops and starts. The destination? A healthier, happier you. Each step you take on this path, no matter how small, is a victory in its own right, bringing you closer to your overall goals.

Managing Stress and Emotional Eating

Tackling stress and emotional eating is like being on a dieting tightrope, where emotions are the winds trying to throw you off balance. It's not just about willpower but about finding the right balance and techniques to keep you steady.

Identifying Emotional Triggers:
Like a detective examining clues, identify what prompts your emotional eating. Is it stress from work, loneliness at night, or even celebration that leads you to overindulge? Recognizing these triggers is like having a map to navigate your emotional landscape. It requires honest self-reflection. Perhaps keeping a food diary can help spot patterns. For instance, you might notice that stress at work leads to late-night snacking or feelings of sadness driving you to comfort foods. This awareness is crucial in developing strategies to manage these emotional eating habits.

Mastering Stress Management:
Imagine your stress as a cluttered desk. Just as you would organize this space, organize your stress management techniques. It could be meditation, likened to filing away anxieties, or yoga, akin to straightening out the papers. These techniques don't eliminate stress, but they help tidy it up. Consider other stress-reduction techniques like deep breathing exercises, engaging in a hobby, or simply taking a walk. The idea is to find what works best for you – it might be listening to music, gardening, or even painting. The goal is to have a go-to activity to help you unwind and distract from the emotional urge to eat.

Alternatives to Eating:

If boredom or loneliness are your triggers, think of activities that are as satisfying as your favorite snack but without the calories. Is reading a book or painting as comforting as a bowl of ice cream? Can a walk be as refreshing as raiding the fridge? These substitutes can keep your hands and mind busy without adding to your waistline.

It's about replacing the habit of reaching for food with something that nourishes you in other ways. It could be calling a friend, writing in a journal, or engaging in a craft. The key is to have these alternatives readily available so that when the urge hits, you have a plan in place.

Embracing Mindful Eating:
Mindful eating is like tunning into a fine radio frequency. It's about really listening to your body and eating with intention and attention. This means savoring each bite and recognizing your body's hunger and fullness signals rather than mindlessly munching while distracted.

Try to eat in a calm environment, free from electronic distractions. Focus on the flavors, textures, and smells of your food. By eating mindfully, you enjoy your food more and naturally eat less, as you're giving your body time to register fullness.

Food and Mood Journaling:
Keeping a journal is like having a daily debrief with yourself. Note what you ate, how you felt before eating, and your feelings afterward. Over time, patterns emerge, offering insights into your eating habits and how they're intertwined with your emotions. This can be a powerful tool in understanding the emotional aspects of your eating habits. It can also help identify healthier dynamic coping mechanisms that don't involve food.

Seeking Professional Guidance:
If emotional eating feels overwhelming, like a ship trying to navigate a storm, consider seeking help from a nutritionist or therapist. They can be the lighthouse guiding you to safer shores. Sometimes, having an expert's perspective can provide new coping

strategies and insights you might not have figured out independently.

Non-Food Rewards:
Develop a reward system that doesn't involve food. Finished a stressful project? How about rewarding yourself with a new book, a movie night, or a relaxing bath? These rewards can act as positive reinforcement for handling stress healthily. Finding joy and satisfaction in accomplishments that don't revolve around food is necessary, reinforcing your journey towards healthier coping mechanisms.

Adopting these coping mechanisms is a process, one that requires patience and persistence. It's about finding the right tools and techniques that work for you, keeping you balanced on the tightrope of healthy eating amidst life's emotional ups and downs. The goal is to develop a relationship with food that is healthy and balanced, where food is seen as nourishment rather than a means to cope with emotions.

Goal Setting: Creating Achievable and Measurable Goals Using the SMART Approach

Embarking on the journey to a healthier lifestyle is like setting sail towards a distant, promising shore. To navigate successfully, you need a well-defined map - this is where SMART goal setting comes in, providing clarity and direction.

S - Specific:

Clarifying the Details:
Goals need to be clear-cut and precise. Think of it as using a GPS; you need an exact destination, not just a general direction.

Application:
Replace "I want to get fit" with "I will engage in 30 minutes of cardio three times a week." It's like deciding not just to read more but to read one book per month.

Example: For healthier eating, rather than a vague "eat better," specify "include a serving of leafy greens in at least two meals daily."

The specificity acts as a clear guide, giving you a concrete target to aim for. It helps measure progress and keeps you focused on the exact task.

M - Measurable:

Tracking Your Journey: A measurable goal allows you to track progress. It's like marking your trail while hiking, so you know how far you've come and how far to go.

Application: "I will drink eight glasses of water daily" is quantifiable, unlike the nebulous "drink more water."

Example: If cutting down on coffee, a measurable goal is to "reduce coffee intake to one cup per day."

Quantifying your goals allows you to see your progress in real numbers, which can be incredibly motivating and provide a sense of accomplishment.

A - Achievable:

Realistic Aspirations:
Goals should stretch your abilities but remain attainable. It's like training for a hill climb before attempting the mountain.
Application: Instead of an unfeasible "lose 30 pounds in a month," aim for "lose 8 pounds in a month."

Example:
If new to exercise, an achievable goal is "start with 10 minutes of daily stretching," rather than immediately aiming for an hour of intense workout.

Setting achievable goals ensures that you're setting yourself up for success, not disappointment. It keeps you motivated and helps build confidence as you meet these realistic targets.

R - Relevant:

Aligning with Your Life:
Your goals should align with your values and larger life plans.
They should feel important to you, like choosing the right gear for
a hiking trip that suits your style.
Application: If family is your focus, a relevant goal could be
"prepare a healthy family meal twice a week."

Example: For stress management, a pertinent goal might be to
"dedicate 15 minutes before bed to relaxation and unwinding."

Relevance ensures that your goals are meaningful to you and fit
well with your overall lifestyle and priorities.

T - Time-Bound:

Setting a Deadline:
Assign a timeframe to your goal for added motivation. It's like
setting a countdown for a launch; it builds anticipation and
urgency.

Application:
"I will increase my daily step count to 10,000 within the next two
months" gives you a clear timeline.

Example:
If trying to improve sleep habits, a time-bound goal is to
"establish a regular sleep schedule by going to bed at 10 PM each
night for the next month."

Adding a time element creates a sense of urgency and can spur you
into action. It helps prevent procrastination and keeps you focused
on the deadline.

By integrating the SMART approach into your goal-setting
process, you transform vague wishes into tangible targets. It's not
just about setting sail; it's about plotting a course, adjusting the
sails correctly, and having a clear destination in sight.

This approach breaks down the overwhelming into manageable chunks, making your health journey both rewarding and achievable. Setting SMART goals turns the abstract into the attainable, providing a clear roadmap on your journey to better health.

Chapter 7: Natural Supplements and Athlete Nutrition

"Natural supplements bridge the gap between nutrition and peak performance, fueling the body for excellence." - Dr. Andrew Weil

Natural supplements have become increasingly popular for those aiming to boost their health and athletic performance. But what are these supplements, and why do they attract so much attention from fitness enthusiasts and professional athletes?

Natural supplements are products designed to complement your diet and provide nutrients, such as vitamins, minerals, amino acids, and enzymes that you may not be getting in sufficient quantities from your meals alone. Imagine you're building a house (your body) and have most of your materials (nutrients from food). Supplements are like the special bricks that could strengthen your house, especially in areas prone to damage or under heavy strain.

While there's no doubt that supplements can offer significant benefits—such as filling nutritional gaps, enhancing energy levels, and supporting recovery from intense physical activity—they're not without their complications. It's like adding a powerful new appliance to your home's electrical system. If not chosen wisely or used correctly, it could cause more issues than it solves.

One key concern is the potential for supplements to interact with medications you're already taking or to cause side effects on their own. For example, certain supplements might increase the risk of bleeding if you're on blood-thinning medication, or they could affect the metabolism of other drugs, altering their effectiveness.

This is why involving your doctor or a healthcare professional in your decision to take supplements is not just wise—it's essential. They can help you navigate the various available supplements, pinpoint which could benefit your health and athletic performance, and advise you on any potential side effects or interactions with your current health regimen.

The whole idea here is to view supplements as allies in your health and fitness journey, capable of providing support where needed. Yet, like any ally, their role and impact must be carefully considered and monitored to ensure they contribute positively to your overall well-being.

Balancing Benefits and Risks

Supplements offer a convenient way to ensure your body gets the nutrients it needs to function optimally. For athletes, certain supplements can be the key to pushing past plateaus, enhancing recovery, and optimizing performance. However, it's not all smooth sailing. Even natural supplements can have side effects; some might interact with prescription medications unexpectedly. For instance, high doses of vitamin C can interfere with the effectiveness of certain heart medications, while supplements like St. John's Wort can reduce the efficacy of birth control pills.

The Importance of Professional Guidance

Just as you wouldn't add a new component to your training regimen without consulting your coach, incorporating supplements into your diet should be done under the guidance of a healthcare professional. They can help you understand which supplements could be beneficial, how to take them safely, and what signs to watch for in case of adverse reactions.

Moreover, healthcare providers can offer insights into how different supplements might interact with each other and with any medications you're taking, ensuring that your supplementation approach is safe and effective.

[80]

Key Supplements for Overall Health and Athletic Performance

Selecting the appropriate supplements is crucial for enhancing your health and athletic performance. Each supplement serves a distinct purpose, uniquely contributing to your well-being. Here, we'll explore some essential supplements recognized for their benefits to athletes and individuals aiming to boost their overall health.

Vitamin D: The Sunshine Vitamin

- **Why It's Important:** Vitamin D plays a vital role in bone health, immune function, and muscle recovery. For athletes, adequate Vitamin D levels are crucial for optimal performance and to decrease the risk of injuries. It's not just about stronger bones; Vitamin D is integral for overall health, supporting everything from heart health to immune responses, making it a powerhouse nutrient for anyone active.

- **How to Get It:** While sunlight is a primary source, living in areas with less sunshine or wearing sunscreen (which blocks Vitamin D synthesis) can lead to deficiencies. Foods like fatty fish and fortified products offer some Vitamin D, but supplements can help fill the gap. When considering supplementation, it's important to choose a form easily absorbed by the body, such as Vitamin D3, and to discuss the appropriate dosage with a healthcare provider.

Magnesium: The Multitasker

- **Why It's Important:** Magnesium supports over 300 biochemical reactions in the body, including muscle and nerve function, energy production, and protein synthesis.

It's particularly beneficial in preventing cramps and aiding recovery post-exercise. Magnesium's role in energy production makes it a critical nutrient for sustaining long workouts and aiding in the recovery process, ensuring that athletes can perform their best day after day.

- **How to Get It:** Green leafy vegetables, nuts, seeds, and whole grains are great sources. However, athletes with high-intensity training routines may require more than the diet alone can provide. This is where supplements come in handy, offering a convenient way to ensure adequate intake. Look for magnesium in forms that are easily absorbed, such as magnesium citrate or glycinate.

Calcium: For Strong Bones and Beyond

- **Why It's Important:** Calcium is well-known for its role in building and maintaining strong bones, which is essential for everyone, athletes included. It also plays a role in muscle function and nerve signaling. This mineral is key for bone health and its critical role in muscle contractions and cardiovascular function, making it essential for sustained physical activity.

- **How to Get It:** Dairy products, leafy greens, and fortified plant-based milk are excellent sources. Supplements can be an option for those with a dairy intolerance or who prefer a plant-based diet. When selecting a calcium supplement, consider one that includes Vitamin D to enhance absorption.

Potassium: The Electrolyte Manager

- **Why It's Important:** Potassium helps regulate fluid balance, muscle contractions, and nerve signals. A critical electrolyte for athletes, it helps prevent muscle cramps and supports cardiovascular health. Its role in fluid balance and nerve function is crucial for maintaining endurance and preventing fatigue during long periods of exercise.

- **How to Get It:** Bananas, potatoes, spinach, and avocados are rich in potassium. During heavy training, supplements can help ensure levels are sufficient. Ensuring adequate potassium intake is especially important for athletes in endurance sports or those training in hot climates, where electrolyte balance is key to preventing dehydration and cramping.

Iron with Vitamin C: The Energy Duo

- **Why it's Important:** Iron is vital for creating hemoglobin, which carries oxygen to your muscles and is crucial for energy and performance. Vitamin C enhances iron absorption, making these two a great team. This combination is especially important for athletes or anyone engaged in regular physical activity, as it supports energy levels and overall endurance.

- **How to Get It:** Combining iron-rich foods like spinach and red meat with Vitamin C-rich foods like oranges or strawberries can boost absorption. Supplements might be necessary for those with identified deficiencies. It's important to consult with a healthcare provider when considering iron supplements, as iron needs can vary widely among individuals.

B Vitamins: The Energy and Recovery Helpers

- **Why they're important:** B vitamins are involved in energy production and the repair of muscle damage from exercise. They're essential for converting food into energy. This group of vitamins is crucial for anyone looking to maintain energy levels through busy days or demanding workouts, supporting everything from the health of red blood cells to energy metabolism.

- **How to Get It:** Whole grains, meats, eggs, and legumes are packed with B vitamins. Athletes, especially those on a vegetarian or vegan diet, might benefit from supplementation to ensure they're getting enough. B-complex supplements can provide a balanced mix of essential B vitamins in convenient forms.

Safe Supplementation Practices

Understanding how to choose and use supplements safely is crucial for maximizing their benefits while minimizing risks. This includes knowing which products are reliable, determining appropriate dosages, and recognizing that more isn't always better.

- **Choosing High-Quality Supplements**

The market is flooded with different kinds of supplements, making it challenging to know which ones are trustworthy. Look for products that have been third-party tested and verified, which means an independent organization has checked them for purity and accuracy in labeling. Certifications from organizations like the U.S. Pharmacopeia (USP) or NSF International are good quality indicators.

- **Understanding Dosages**

The Recommended Dietary Allowances (RDAs) are a great starting point to understand how much of each nutrient you need daily. However, individual needs can vary based on age, sex, health status, and physical activity level. It's very important to read supplement labels carefully and discuss them with a healthcare provider to tailor dosages to your needs.

- **Avoiding Interactions and Side Effects**

Supplements can interact with medications, other supplements, and even foods, sometimes causing harmful effects. For example,

[84]

high doses of vitamin E can increase the risk of bleeding, especially if you're taking blood-thinning medications. Sharing all the supplements and medications you're taking with your healthcare provider can help prevent adverse interactions.

The Role of Healthcare Providers

A healthcare provider can offer personalized advice based on your health history, dietary habits, and lifestyle. They can also monitor for side effects and adjust dosages as needed. This partnership is key to using supplements effectively and safely.

- **Listening to Your Body**

Pay attention to how your body responds after you start taking a supplement. If you notice any new symptoms or changes, such as digestive upset, skin rashes, or changes in energy levels, consult your healthcare provider. These could be signs that a supplement isn't right for you or that the dosage needs adjustment.

Supplements and a Balanced Diet

It's essential to understand that supplements are designed to complement, not replace, the nutrients you get from whole foods. A balanced diet rich in fruits, vegetables, whole grains, lean proteins, and healthy fats offers various nutrients, fiber, and antioxidants fundamental for your health. These whole foods provide a complex nutritional profile that supplements alone cannot replicate, serving as the cornerstone of any effective health and wellness strategy.

While adding supplements to your routine, it's important to approach this as a strategic enhancement to an already nutritious diet. The goal is to use supplements to fill nutritional gaps and bolster your intake of certain nutrients, particularly in areas where your regular diet might not suffice. For example, if you have a known deficiency in a specific vitamin or mineral or dietary restrictions limit your intake of certain nutrients, supplements can provide a crucial boost to ensure your body gets everything it needs to function optimally.

However, it's crucial to remember that supplements are just one component of a broader health and wellness framework. Physical activity, stress management, getting enough sleep, and a balanced diet all contribute to your overall well-being.

Supplements are intended to support and enhance these lifestyle factors, not replace them. By thoughtfully integrating supplements into a well-rounded diet and lifestyle, you can create a comprehensive approach to health that supports your body's needs and helps you achieve your wellness goals.

Reflecting Your Journey with Supplements

- What are the natural supplements you're currently taking, if any? List them down and research their benefits and potential side effects.

- Considering your daily diet, identify potential nutritional gaps. Could any specific supplements help fill these gaps?

Exercise – Personal Supplement Plan:

- Based on what you've learned, draft a simple supplement plan that aligns with your health and fitness goals. Remember, the aim is not to rely solely on supplements but to use them strategically to complement your diet.

- Schedule a consultation with a healthcare provider to discuss your draft supplement plan. It's crucial to ensure that any supplements you consider are safe and beneficial for you, especially in relation to any health conditions or medications you might be taking.

Chapter 8: The Role of Appetite Suppressants in Weight Loss

"Controlling appetite is not about denying hunger but learning to understand and manage it." - Dr. Yoni Freedhoff.

Appetite suppressants are tools designed to help control hunger and reduce food cravings, making it easier for individuals to manage their eating habits and support weight loss efforts. They come in various forms, including *prescription medications, over-the-counter supplements, and natural methods* that rely on specific foods or eating practices.

The principle behind appetite suppressants is straightforward: by diminishing the sensation of hunger or making you feel full sooner, these methods can help you consume fewer calories throughout the day. This can be particularly useful for those who find their hunger cues or cravings challenging to manage with diet and exercise alone.

Prescription appetite suppressants are typically used under medical supervision, especially for individuals with obesity or related health conditions. These medications are potent tools but are generally recommended for short-term use due to potential side effects and the risk of dependence.

On the other hand, **over-the-counter supplements** that claim to suppress appetite might include ingredients like dietary fiber, which increases the feeling of fullness; green tea extract, known for its metabolic benefits; and caffeine, which can reduce the perception of hunger. While these supplements can offer some assistance, their effectiveness can vary widely. Not all are backed by strong scientific evidence. Therefore, it's crucial to approach these options cautiously and, ideally, under the guidance of a healthcare professional.

Natural appetite suppressants involve consuming foods high in fiber and protein, which promote satiety, or adopting habits that help control hunger, such as drinking plenty of water and focusing on mindful eating. These methods can be effective, safe ways to support weight management without needing medication or supplements.

Regardless of the method chosen, it's important to remember that appetite suppressants should complement a healthy lifestyle, including a balanced diet and regular physical activity, rather than replace them. They can be valuable tools in achieving weight management goals, but they work best when used as part of a comprehensive approach to health.

Prescription Medications for Appetite Suppression:

- Prescription medications designed to suppress appetite play a significant role in the treatment of obesity and related health conditions. These medications, such as phentermine, are often part of a comprehensive weight-loss plan that includes diet, exercise, and behavioral changes.

- Their primary function is to reduce hunger sensations or make you feel full faster during meals, which can help decrease overall calorie intake. Doctors typically prescribe these medications for short-term use, recognizing that the long-term solution to weight management lies in lifestyle modifications. The effectiveness of prescription appetite suppressants varies from person to person, with some experiencing significant benefits in their weight loss journey while others may see more modest results.

- It's crucial to use these medications under the strict guidance of a healthcare professional. They can assess whether a prescription appetite suppressant is appropriate based on your health history, weight loss needs, and potential risk factors. Regular check-ups are essential to monitor your progress and any side effects you might experience. Common side effects can include dry mouth, increased heart rate, and insomnia, though these vary by medication and individual.

Over-the-Counter Supplements: A Closer Look

- The shelves of health stores and pharmacies are lined with over-the-counter (OTC) supplements claiming to suppress appetite and support weight loss. These supplements often contain ingredients like dietary fiber, green tea extract, or caffeine, each purporting to offer a shortcut to shedding pounds by curbing hunger and enhancing metabolism. However, navigating these claims requires a discerning eye and a dose of skepticism.

- Dietary fiber supplements, for instance, can help increase feelings of fullness, potentially leading you to eat less throughout the day. Similarly, green tea extract is touted for its metabolic benefits, possibly giving you a slight edge in calorie burning. Caffeine, known for its stimulant properties, may reduce appetite temporarily. Yet, the effectiveness of these supplements can vary widely among individuals, and their long-term benefits and safety are not always guaranteed.

- Before reaching for an OTC appetite suppressant, it's wise to consider its potential impact on your health and weight loss efforts. Unlike prescription medications, the regulation of dietary supplements is less strict, meaning the quality and concentration of ingredients can differ significantly from one product to another. This variability makes it challenging to predict how effective or safe an OTC supplement will be without proper testing and verification.

Consulting with a healthcare professional is crucial before incorporating any appetite-suppressant supplement into your routine. A doctor or nutritionist can provide valuable insights into whether a supplement could benefit you, considering your overall health, dietary habits, and weight loss goals.

Relying solely on supplements without addressing the foundational aspects of a healthy lifestyle—such as a balanced diet and regular exercise—is unlikely to yield lasting results. Supplements might support your weight management plan, but they are not a magic solution.

Natural Appetite Suppressants: Foods and Practices

- Turning to nature offers a variety of ways to manage appetite without the need for pills or potions. Certain foods and eating habits naturally promote feelings of fullness and can help keep those nagging hunger pangs at bay. Integrating these natural appetite suppressants into your daily routine can support your weight management goals healthily and sustainably.

- High-fiber foods are excellent at making you feel full and satisfied. Fruits, vegetables, whole grains, and legumes contain dietary fiber, slowing digestion and increasing the feeling of fullness for longer periods. Including these foods in your meals can naturally reduce your food intake without leaving you feeling deprived.

- Proteins also play a crucial role in satiety. Foods rich in protein, such as lean meats, fish, eggs, dairy, and plant-based alternatives like tofu and legumes, help maintain muscle mass and keep you feeling full longer. Incorporating a protein source in each meal can effectively manage your hunger levels and reduce the likelihood of snacking on less healthy options.

- Hydration is another key element in appetite control. Sometimes, the body can mistake thirst for hunger. Drinking adequate water throughout the day can help prevent this confusion, reducing unnecessary snacking. Starting a meal with a glass of water is a simple practice that can aid in feeling more satiated and potentially eating less. Additionally, foods with high water content, such as soups, salads, and fruits like watermelon and oranges, contribute to fullness and hydration without adding a significant calorie load.

- Eating slowly is a mindful practice that encourages better digestion and increases the likelihood of feeling full. It takes about 20 minutes for the brain to register that the stomach is full. By slowing down, you give your body the chance to recognize fullness, reducing the chance of overeating. This can be as simple as putting down your utensils between bites or chewing your food more thoroughly.

- Lastly, managing stress and getting adequate sleep are crucial practices that indirectly influence appetite control. Stress and sleep deprivation can lead to hormonal imbalances that increase hunger and cravings, particularly for high-calorie, sugary, and fatty foods. Engaging in stress-reducing activities, such as exercise, meditation, or hobbies, and prioritizing good sleep hygiene can help maintain hormonal balance and support appetite regulation.

Combining Appetite Suppressants with a Healthy Lifestyle

Integrating appetite suppressants into your life, whether prescription medications, over-the-counter supplements, or natural methods, is just one piece of the puzzle in achieving a healthier, more balanced lifestyle. These tools can support managing hunger and cravings, but they deliver the best results when used in conjunction with a comprehensive approach to wellness that includes nutritious eating, regular physical activity, and adequate rest.

A balanced diet rich in fruits, vegetables, whole grains, lean proteins, and healthy fats provides the body with essential nutrients for optimal health and energy. This nutritional foundation supports the body's needs, allowing any form of appetite suppressant to function more effectively by complementing an already healthy diet, rather than trying to compensate for poor eating habits.

Regular physical activity is another cornerstone of a healthy lifestyle that works hand in hand with appetite management. Exercise helps burn calories and build muscle and can positively affect hunger hormones, reducing the urge to overeat. Additionally, the psychological benefits of exercise, including stress reduction and improved mood, can decrease the likelihood of emotional eating.

Adequate rest and stress management are equally important in supporting a balanced approach to appetite control. Ultimately, the goal is to create a sustainable lifestyle supporting weight management and health. Appetite suppressants can be valuable tools in this process, but they are most effective when used as part of a broader strategy that addresses all aspects of health.

Potential Risks and Considerations

Prescription Appetite Suppressants

- Need for vigilance due to potential side effects such as increased heart rate, insomnia, and gastrointestinal disturbances.
- Importance of healthcare professional oversight to monitor for adverse effects and adjust treatment as necessary.

Over-the-Counter Supplements

- Less stringent regulatory environment compared to prescription drugs, leading to variability in product quality and efficacy.
- Risk of supplements containing undisclosed ingredients that could interact with medications or cause side effects.
- Importance of choosing products that have been independently tested and verified for quality.

Natural Appetite Suppressants

- It is generally safer but requires thoughtful integration into diet and routine.
- Risk of overreliance on specific foods for appetite suppression leading to dietary deficiencies.
- Potential health consequences of adopting practices like excessive water intake without proper management.

Overall Strategy for Appetite Suppression

- It should be approached as one component of a broader health and wellness strategy.

- The strategy should include balanced nutrition, physical activity, adequate rest, and stress management.
- The value of open and ongoing dialogue with healthcare providers to tailor an approach that safely and effectively meets individual health goals and needs.

Terpizipide and Semaglutide

"Tirzepatide and Semaglutide" are both significant advancements in the management of weight loss, offering new hope for individuals looking to control their appetite and achieve sustainable weight loss. These medications work by influencing the body's natural signals for hunger and fullness, helping to reduce appetite and extend feelings of satiety. This can lead to a decrease in overall calorie intake, which is crucial for weight loss.

Clinical trials have demonstrated the effectiveness of both tirzepatide and semaglutide. They are part of a class of medications that act on the body's GLP-1 receptor, which plays a key role in regulating hunger. By enhancing the body's response to this receptor, these medications can make managing portion sizes and reducing snacking easier, supporting overall weight loss efforts.

Both medications are administered via subcutaneous injections, which can be conveniently incorporated into a weight management plan.

It's important to approach these treatments under the guidance of a healthcare professional, who can provide personalized advice based on an individual's health history and weight loss goals. As with any medical treatment, a comprehensive approach that includes diet, exercise, and lifestyle changes, in addition to medication, is essential for achieving the best results in weight management.

Chapter 9: The Role of Sleep and Stress Management

"Sleep is the golden chain that ties health and our bodies together." - Thomas Dekker

The relationship between sleep and weight is complex yet fundamentally important for anyone looking to manage their weight effectively. Two hormones are key players here: **leptin and ghrelin**. Leptin, often called the "satiety hormone," signals to your brain that you have enough energy stored and helps regulate appetite. Conversely, ghrelin is known as the "hunger hormone" and stimulates appetite, prompting you to eat. When you're sleep-deprived, your body produces more ghrelin and less leptin, leading to increased hunger and appetite, making weight management more challenging.

Beyond hormonal shifts, lack of sleep also impacts your body's insulin sensitivity, an essential factor in how your body processes sugar. Reduced insulin sensitivity can lead to higher blood sugar levels and increased fat storage, further complicating efforts to maintain or lose weight. This disruption of blood sugar control underscores the importance of quality sleep in maintaining metabolic health and preventing conditions such as obesity and diabetes.

The body's circadian rhythm, or internal clock, is critical in weight management. This natural cycle regulates feelings of sleepiness and wakefulness over 24 hours. It is influenced by factors such as light exposure and eating patterns. Disruptions to the circadian rhythm, such as those caused by irregular sleep schedules or exposure to light at night, can affect hormone production and appetite regulation, further illustrating the intricate link between sleep and weight.

Understanding these biological connections and highlights is important - why sleep is not just a passive state of rest but an active period crucial for health and well-being, including weight management.

Quality Sleep Strategies: Tips for Better Sleep Hygiene

Achieving quality sleep is essential for not only managing weight but also for overall health and well-being. Sleep hygiene refers to the practices and habits that can create the conditions for good quality sleep. By optimizing your sleep environment and routines, you can enhance sleep quality and duration, which in turn supports hormonal balance, appetite regulation, and weight management.

- **Establish a Consistent Sleep Schedule:** Going to bed and waking up at the same times each day, including weekends, helps regulate your body's internal clock, the circadian rhythm. This consistency makes it easier to fall asleep and wake up naturally, improving sleep quality.

- **Create a Restful Environment:** Your bedroom should be a sleep sanctuary. Keep it cool, quiet, and dark. Use blackout curtains, eye masks, and earplugs to block out light and noise. Ensuring your mattress and pillows are comfortable can also significantly affect your sleep quality.

- **Limit Exposure to Light before Bedtime:** Exposure to light, especially blue light from screens, can interfere with your body's production of melatonin, a hormone that signals your body it's time to sleep. Reducing screen time at least an hour before bed and using warm, dim lighting can help your body prepare for sleep.

- **Mind Your Intake:** Avoiding caffeine and heavy meals in the hours leading up to bedtime can prevent sleep disruptions. While a small, light snack can be okay, heavy or rich foods can lead to discomfort and make it harder to fall asleep. Similarly, while alcohol might make you feel drowsy, it can interfere with the sleep cycle, impacting sleep quality.

- **Establish a Pre-Sleep Routine:** Calming activities before bed can signal your body that it's time to wind down. This might include reading, taking a warm bath, or practicing relaxation exercises. A consistent pre-sleep routine helps ease the transition into sleep.

- **Stay Active During the Day:** Regular physical activity can help you fall asleep faster and enjoy deeper sleep. However, timing is important. Exercise stimulates the body and can make it harder to fall asleep if done too close to bedtime.

Now, let's see how you can put these insights into action and truly make sleep and stress management an important part of your weight management journey. Here are some reflections, questions, and practical tips to help you move forward:

Deep Dive into Your Sleep Patterns:

- Reflect on your current sleep habits. Are you giving yourself enough time to wind down before bed?

- How often do you find yourself using electronic devices right before sleep? Could this be impacting the quality of your rest?

Creating Your Ideal Sleep Sanctuary:

- Take a moment to assess your sleeping environment. Is there anything you can adjust to make it more conducive to restful sleep? Perhaps it's as simple as investing in blackout curtains or maybe it's time for a more comfortable pillow.

Exercise for Better Sleep:

Consider your physical activity levels throughout the day. How can you adjust your exercise routine to enhance your sleep quality?

Remember, the goal is to be active enough that your body is ready to rest at night, but not so stimulated that you're tossing and turning.

Connect and Share:

Share your sleep and stress management goals with a friend or family member. Encourage each other to implement one or two of the strategies mentioned above and check in at the end of the week to share progress and insights.

By actively engaging with these practices and reflections, you're not just aiming for better sleep; you're taking significant steps towards a healthier, more balanced lifestyle that supports your weight management goals and overall well-being.

Stress and Weight: Understanding the Connection

D id you know that stress can sneak up on you and add extra pounds without realizing it? It's true! When life gets stressful, it can mess with your weight in ways you might not expect. Let's closely examine how stress impacts your body weight and some tips to fight back.

First, let's talk about cortisol — the stress hormone your body releases when you're feeling the pressure. Cortisol is like the body's alarm system, but when it's constantly ringing because of ongoing stress, it can lead to weight gain. Why? Because it ramps up your hunger for those oh-so-comforting but high-calorie snacks like sweets and fatty foods. Plus, it has a sneaky way of storing fat around your belly, which is not only frustrating but also not good for your health.

Stress doesn't just mess with your hormones; it can also destroy your healthy habits.

Have you ever found yourself too stressed to cook and opted for takeout instead? Or too drained to even think about going for a run or hitting the gym? You're not alone. Stress can make it tough to stick to your eating plan and stay active, leading you to a more sedentary lifestyle.
And let's not forget about sleep. Stress and sleep are like rivals; when one goes up, the other tends to go down. Poor sleep can make stress feel even worse, and when you're not sleeping well, your body's appetite hormones get all out of whack. This can make you feel hungrier and sabotage your efforts to manage your weight.

So, what can you do about it? First, recognize that stress might be part of the reason managing your weight feels like an uphill battle.

Next, start looking for ways to dial down the stress in your life. Whether it's getting more active, trying out some relaxation techniques, making sure you're getting enough sleep, or reaching out to friends, family, or a pro for a chat — there are lots of strategies that can help keep stress (and its impact on your weight) in check.

Remember, understanding how stress affects your weight is a powerful first step. From there, small changes to manage stress better can make a big difference in reaching your health and weight goals. You've got this!

Relaxation Techniques: Mindfulness, Meditation, and Yoga

As you have seen, battling stress is key to managing weight effectively. Including relaxation practices like mindfulness, meditation, and yoga in your day can make a big difference. These aren't just good for your mind; they have real benefits for your body, helping you handle the stress that can lead to putting on pounds.

Mindfulness:
This involves bringing your attention to the present moment, observing your thoughts, feelings, and bodily sensations without judgment. This practice can be applied to eating, known as mindful eating, where you pay close attention to the experience of eating, savor each bite, and tune into your body's hunger and fullness cues. Mindful eating can prevent overeating by enhancing your awareness of when and why you eat, leading to more deliberate and satisfying food choices.

Practical Action Tips:
- Start by dedicating a few minutes each day to sit quietly and focus on your breath or a specific object.
- Practice eating without distractions like TV or smartphones, focusing on your food's flavors, textures, and aromas.
- Use mindfulness apps or guided sessions to help develop your practice.

Meditation:

This practice of concentrated focus aims to quiet the mind and induce a calm state. Regular meditation can lower cortisol levels, reducing the urge to eat in response to stress. It can also improve sleep quality, further supporting weight management efforts.

Practical Action Tips:

- Set aside a regular time each day for meditation, starting with just 5-10 minutes.
- Find a quiet, comfortable place where you won't be disturbed.
- Use guided meditation recordings or apps designed for beginners to help you get started.

Yoga:

Yoga combines physical postures, breath control, and meditation to enhance physical flexibility, reduce stress, and promote relaxation. Yoga can be particularly effective in managing stress-related weight gain, as it addresses the mental and emotional aspects of stress and provides a form of physical exercise.

Practical Action Tips:

- Join a beginner's yoga class to learn proper techniques and postures.
- Incorporate yoga into your routine at least 2-3 times weekly for noticeable benefits.
- Explore different styles of yoga to find the one that best suits your needs and preferences.

Adding mindfulness, meditation, and yoga to your life offers a strong defense against the stress that can mess with your weight goals. These practices promote peace and well-being, making your journey to managing weight smoother and more positive.

Chapter 10: Building a Support System

"Alone we can do so little; together we can do so much." –
Helen Keller.

The journey to better health, weight management, or any personal growth goal must not be solitary. In fact, research shows that having a supportive community can significantly enhance your chances of success. Supportive relationships provide motivation, accountability, and encouragement, which are invaluable when facing challenges or setbacks.

Why Social Support?

Studies have demonstrated that individuals with strong social support networks have better health outcomes, including more effective weight management. Supportive communities can provide emotional encouragement, practical advice, and shared experiences that are crucial in your weight loss journey.

Finding Your Community

Discovering a community that aligns with your goals and values might seem daunting, but there are more opportunities than ever to connect with like-minded individuals. This can include joining fitness or wellness groups, participating in local health-oriented classes, or becoming part of online forums dedicated to similar objectives. The key is to engage in environments that foster positivity and shared goals.

Fostering a Supportive Environment

Once you find a community, actively participating and contributing to the supportive environment is crucial. Sharing your experiences, challenges, and successes not only helps you but also motivates and inspires others in the community. It's a reciprocal relationship; your support often returns to you manifold.

Harnessing the Power of Social Media

Social media platforms have revolutionized how we connect with others who share our interests and goals. From Facebook groups and Instagram communities to forums and dedicated health apps, there's a vast array of options to explore. These platforms can provide daily inspiration, practical advice, and a sense of belonging, making the journey less isolating. I've found that following hashtags related to my health goals or joining specific challenge groups can introduce me to new ideas, keep me accountable, and uplift me on tough days.

Remember, a supportive community acts as a catalyst for maintaining motivation and perseverance. Whether celebrating achievements or offering a listening ear during tough times, the community around you can be a powerful force for staying on track. Additionally, community involvement can enhance your sense of belonging and purpose, further fueling your motivation.

Role of Healthcare Providers

Navigating your path to better health is a journey that benefits greatly from knowledgeable companions— *"healthcare providers"*. These professionals aren't just sources of treatment or advice; they're partners in crafting a plan that respects your needs, goals, and circumstances.

The Personal Touch

In my experience and years of practice, the relationship with healthcare providers is most effective when it's a partnership. It's not just about presenting symptoms and receiving advice, but a dialogue where your personal health goals are considered, and your treatment or wellness plan is tailored to fit you perfectly. This partnership can offer medical support and emotional encouragement, making the journey towards health less daunting.

Expert Guidance

Healthcare providers bring a wealth of knowledge and expertise to the table. They can help decipher the complex information surrounding health, nutrition, and exercise, offering clear, actionable advice. Whether it's discussing the nuances of a balanced diet, the best exercise regimen for your specific situation, or the safe use of supplements, their input can be invaluable. They can also help monitor progress, adjusting plans to ensure the best outcomes.

A Holistic Approach

The best healthcare providers look at the whole picture, not just isolated issues. They understand that mental health, stress levels, sleep quality, and physical activity influence overall health. Considering all these factors, they can help devise a comprehensive approach that addresses every aspect of well-being.

Finding the Right Provider

The key to a fruitful partnership is finding a healthcare provider who listens, understands, and respects your health goals. This might mean seeking out specialists in certain areas or looking for professionals with a holistic approach to health. Don't hesitate to advocate for yourself and seek out a provider with whom you feel a genuine connection and who supports your journey toward better health.

Engagement and Advocacy
Engaging actively in this partnership means being open about your goals, challenges, and successes. It also means asking questions and seeking clarity on any advice given. Remember, you're the most important advocate for your health, and your engagement can drive the partnership forward.

Family and Friends: Engaging Loved Ones in Your Journey
Embarking on a health and wellness journey is a deeply personal endeavor, yet it's one that flourishes with the support of those closest to us. Family and friends provide a foundational layer of emotional support and play an active role in our pursuit of healthier lifestyles. Engaging our loved ones in this journey can amplify our efforts, making the path less daunting and more joyous. Here are key reasons why you need your family support:

- **The Strength of Emotional Support:** The encouragement and understanding from your family and friends can be a powerful motivator. They're the ones who know us best, cheering us on through victories and offering comfort during setbacks. Their belief in our abilities can sometimes push us to keep going when our motivation wanes.

- **Transforming Activities into Shared Experiences:** Incorporating family and friends into health-related activities can transform these endeavors from solitary tasks into enjoyable shared experiences. Whether preparing a healthy meal together, embarking on weekend hiking adventures, or joining a group fitness class, these activities can strengthen bonds while promoting a healthier lifestyle.

The joy found in these shared moments enriches your relationships and health goals.

- **Navigating Challenges Together:** It's important to acknowledge that involving loved ones in your health journey can also present challenges. Differences in goals, interests, and commitment levels can lead to friction. Open communication is key in these situations. Discussing your goals, the reasons behind them, and how important their support is to you can help align expectations and foster a supportive environment. Remember, it's about finding common ground and mutual respect for each other's journeys.

- **Creating a Supportive Home Environment:** For those sharing a living space with family or roommates, creating an environment that supports healthy choices can have a significant impact. This might mean stocking the kitchen with nutritious food options, establishing shared wellness goals, or even setting collective boundaries around screen time or sleep schedules. When everyone's on board, making healthier choices becomes a seamless part of daily life.

The Ripple Effect of Positive Influence

One of the most beautiful aspects of involving loved ones in your health journey is the potential for positive influence. Your commitment can inspire those around you to reflect on their own health and wellness goals. This reciprocal inspiration creates a cycle of positive change within your circle, reinforcing the idea that together, we can achieve more than we can alone.

Chapter 11: Overcoming Challenges and Setbacks

"Strength does not come from what you can do. It comes from overcoming the things you once thought you couldn't." – Rikki Rogers.

In your pursuit to conquer obesity and to flourish in better health, facing obstacles is inevitable. Challenges are a natural part of the journey, whether they're tied to your emotions, physical condition, or social situations. Acknowledging these hurdles is the first step towards overcoming them, equipping you with the insights to move forward with confidence and resilience.

Emotional Challenges:
Your mindset plays a crucial role in your wellness journey. Feelings of doubt, frustration, or lack of motivation are common emotional hurdles. It's natural to experience days when your goals feel out of reach or when your progress seems too slow. These emotions can stem from internal pressures or comparisons to others' journeys on social media. Remember, your path is unique, and it's okay to have ups and downs.

Physical Challenges:
Physical setbacks, such as injuries, illness, or plateaus in weight loss, can disrupt your progress. These challenges can be particularly disheartening, especially if they limit your ability to engage in activities you enjoy or follow your planned routine. It's important to listen to your body and seek professional advice to address these issues safely.

Social Challenges:
Your social environment can also pose challenges, from well-meaning friends and family who inadvertently undermine your efforts to social situations that tempt you away from your goals. Navigating these situations requires balancing staying true to your goals and maintaining your social relationships.

Facing These Hurdles Head-On

- First, acknowledge that these challenges are a normal part of the journey. You're not alone in facing them, and they do not define your capability or worth.

- Cultivate self-compassion. Be kind to yourself on difficult days and recognize your effort, not just your achievements.

- Communicate your needs and goals with loved ones. Often, they can offer support in ways you hadn't considered.

- Finally, remember the power of resilience. Each hurdle you overcome is a testament to your strength and brings you one step closer to your goals.

Your journey to wellness is a unique experience, including the challenges you meet and overcome along the way. These hurdles, while daunting, are not insurmountable. With perseverance, support, and a bit of creativity, you can navigate these obstacles and continue moving forward.

Strategies for Resilience: Bouncing Back from Setbacks

Developing resilience is like building a muscle; it strengthens through practice and persistence. When faced with setbacks on your health and wellness journey, resilience is the force that propels you forward, transforming challenges into opportunities for growth. Here are strategies to cultivate resilience and bounce back stronger:

- **Adjust Your Perspective:** It's natural to feel discouraged by setbacks, but shifting your perspective can change how you experience them. Instead of seeing a setback as a failure, view it as a learning opportunity. Ask yourself, "What can this experience teach me?" This mindset encourages growth and resilience.

- **Set Realistic Goals and Expectations:** Part of bouncing back involves setting achievable goals that motivate rather than overwhelm. Break your larger goals into smaller, manageable steps. Celebrate each accomplishment, no matter how small, to maintain momentum and motivation.

- **Develop a Support Network:** Surrounding yourself with a supportive community can significantly impact your ability to overcome challenges. Whether it's family, friends, or online support groups, a network of encouragement and advice can provide the strength needed to persist.

- **Practice Self-Care:** Resilience is not just about pushing through obstacles; it's also about knowing when to rest and recharge. Prioritize activities that nourish your body and mind, such as adequate sleep, nutritious food, physical activity, and relaxation techniques. Self-care reinforces your mental and physical resources, enabling you to effectively tackle challenges.

- **Learn Stress Management Techniques:** In the earlier chapters, we discussed stress management in detail. Effective stress management is crucial for resilience. Techniques such as mindfulness, deep breathing, and meditation can help you stay centered and calm, even in the face of setbacks. Incorporating these practices into your daily routine can improve your ability to respond to challenges with flexibility and strength.

- **Seek Professional Guidance When Needed:** Sometimes, the best way to bounce back is with the help of a professional. Professional guidance can offer valuable insights and strategies tailored to your personal journey, whether you're a counselor, coach, or healthcare provider.

Remember, resilience is not about avoiding setbacks but how you respond to them. By embracing resilience-building strategies, you equip yourself with the tools to navigate the ups and downs of your health and wellness journey. Each setback is an opportunity to learn, grow, and emerge stronger on the other side.

Long-term Perspective: Keeping the End Goal in Sight

It's important to focus on your long-term health goals, understanding that the journey to managing weight and overcoming obesity is a marathon, not a sprint. There will be ups and downs, but keeping your ultimate goals in mind helps you move forward with determination. Remember, real progress comes from lasting changes, not quick fixes.

1) **Embrace Patience and Persistence**: The path to better health requires patience. Changes, especially those related to weight and lifestyle, don't happen overnight. They unfold through consistent effort over time. Remind yourself that every choice you make contributes to your long-term success. This mindset helps in maintaining focus, especially when short-term progress seems slow.

2) **Adjust and Adapt**: A long-term perspective also means being flexible and willing to adjust your strategies as needed. What works well at one stage of your journey might need tweaking later. Regularly reassess your goals, strategies, and progress. Being open to change ensures your approach aligns with your evolving needs and circumstances.

3) **Visualize Success**: Visualization is a powerful tool. Regularly take time to visualize yourself achieving your goals. How does it feel to live in a healthier body? What activities are you enjoying? Visualization reinforces your commitment and makes your goals feel more tangible and attainable.

4) **Stay Educated and Informed**: Knowledge is power. Stay informed about health, nutrition, and wellness. Understanding the science behind weight management and health can bolster your commitment to your goals,

helping you make informed choices that support your long-term success.

Keeping the end goal in sight means recognizing that health and wellness are lifelong pursuits.

Your journey is about more than just reaching a specific number on the scale—it's about building a life where healthy choices are woven into the fabric of your daily existence, bringing you closer to your vision of health and happiness.

Celebrating Milestones: Recognizing and Celebrating Progress

Acknowledging and celebrating your progress is not just a rewarding part of your health journey; it's a vital one. Each milestone reached, no matter how small it might seem, is a testament to your dedication, effort, and growth. These moments of celebration breathe life into your journey, reinforcing your motivation and commitment to your goals:

Recognizing Your Progress
First, it's important to recognize all types of progress, not just the numbers on the scale. Did you make it through a tough workout? Have you found yourself reaching for water instead of soda more often? Maybe you've noticed an improvement in how you feel physically or emotionally. All these are milestones worthy of recognition. They reflect changes in your behavior and mindset crucial for long-term success.

Setting Up a Milestone Tracker
Creating a tangible way to track and celebrate your milestones can make this process even more enjoyable. Here's a simple game plan to get started:

- Create a Milestone Board: Use a corkboard, whiteboard, or digital app to track your progress visually. Include both big goals and small steps.

- Use Visual Markers: For each goal or milestone, place a visual marker like a sticker, pin, or digital icon. Choose something that brings you joy and satisfaction to add.

- Incorporate Rewards: Decide on a reward for each milestone you achieve. Rewards should be motivating and aligned with your wellness goals—think a massage, a new book, or a day trip to a place you love.

- Share Your Achievements: Consider sharing your milestones with your support network. This can amplify your sense of achievement and allow those who support you to celebrate your successes alongside you.

- Reflect and Reset: Once you've celebrated a milestone, reflect on what you've learned and how you've grown. Then, set your sights on the next goal, adjusting your game plan as needed.

Celebration as Motivation
Remember, the act of celebrating isn't just about giving yourself a pat on the back; it's about reinforcing the behaviors and choices that got you to this point. It's a way to remind yourself why you started this journey and to fuel your motivation for the challenges ahead.

Let these celebrations be reminders of how far you've come and the incredible potential you have to continue moving forward. The path to wellness is a journey of a thousand steps, and each one is a reason to celebrate.

Chapter 12: future Trends in Obesity and Lifestyle Medicine

"Innovation in health means tailoring prevention, not just treatment. The future is personalized." - Dr. David Katz

We are at a turning point with new discoveries and methods for tackling obesity and enhancing lifestyle medicine. It's a thrilling moment to witness and be part of these advancements. The upcoming years promise more tailored and effective ways to handle and prevent obesity, a growing challenge globally. Adapting to these changes means understanding the new directions and innovative strategies that will redefine how we approach obesity management.

Personalized Medicine in Obesity Management

The future of obesity management is shifting towards a more personalized approach, where treatments and lifestyle interventions are tailored specifically to you. Imagine a scenario where a simple genetic test could reveal the most effective diet for your body type or where an analysis of your microbiome—the community of microorganisms living in your gut—could guide personalized nutrition plans that help manage your weight more effectively.

This tailored approach extends beyond nutrition to encompass all facets of lifestyle medicine, including physical activity and mental health strategies. Advances in understanding the human genome and microbiome are paving the way for interventions that are not one-size-fits-all but are instead customized to your unique genetic makeup and lifestyle.

The Role of Genetics and Metabolism

Your genes play a significant role in determining how your body processes food, your predisposition to certain types of exercise, and even your likelihood of developing obesity-related conditions. By analyzing your genetic profile, healthcare providers can predict which lifestyle changes and treatments will be most effective for you, reducing the trial-and-error approach that often makes weight management frustrating.

Technological Innovations and Digital Health

The role of technology in managing health and wellness, especially in the context of obesity, is expanding rapidly. Wearables, mobile apps, and digital platforms are not just gadgets and software; they are becoming essential tools in our health management toolkit. These technologies offer new ways to monitor your health, keep track of your progress, and stay motivated.

- **Wearables and Mobile Apps:** Imagine having a personal health coach with you at all times, one that tracks your steps, monitors your heart rate, analyzes your sleep patterns, and even reminds you to hydrate and stand up after long periods of sitting. That's the power of wearable technology. Similarly, mobile apps can help you log your food intake, plan your workouts, and connect with a community for support and inspiration. These tools make it easier to stay on top of your health goals by providing real-time feedback and personalized insights.

The Psychological Dimension of Obesity

Addressing obesity requires more than just focusing on physical health; it involves understanding and managing the psychological factors contributing to weight gain and hindering weight loss. Techniques like cognitive behavioral therapy (CBT) and other psychological interventions are gaining recognition for their effectiveness in tackling the mental and emotional challenges associated with obesity.

- **Cognitive Behavioral Therapy (CBT):** CBT is a form of therapy that helps you become aware of inaccurate or negative thinking so you can view challenging situations more clearly and respond to them more effectively. For managing obesity, CBT can help you identify and change behaviors and thought patterns that contribute to unhealthy eating habits, lack of exercise, and weight gain. It teaches strategies for coping with cravings, setting realistic goals, and dealing with setbacks positively.

- **Addressing Emotional Eating:** One of the key psychological challenges in obesity is emotional eating — the tendency to respond to stress, anxiety, or other emotions by eating, often unhealthily. Recognizing the triggers of emotional eating is the first step in addressing it. Techniques learned in CBT, mindfulness practices, and stress management strategies can help you find healthier ways to cope with emotions without turning to food.

- **Building a Positive Self-Image:** Another important aspect is building a positive self-image and breaking the cycle of negative self-talk and guilt often associated with obesity. This includes learning to appreciate your body for what it can do rather than focusing solely on appearance or weight. Celebrating small achievements and focusing on non-weight-related health improvements can boost self-esteem and motivation.

The Promise of Personalized Nutrition

The concept of personalized nutrition, where dietary recommendations are tailored to an individual's genetic makeup, lifestyle, and health status, is gaining traction.

Advances in genomics and metabolomics—the study of metabolic processes—offer insights into how we can optimize our diets for weight management and overall health. In the future, we may see nutrition plans as unique as our DNA, maximizing the effectiveness of diet in preventing and managing obesity.

Conclufion

Congratulations on reaching the final page of this transformative journey. It's far from just the close of a book; it's the dawn of a new chapter in your life—a chapter where prioritizing your health and happiness is paramount. This book has been a map, guiding you through the complexities of managing weight and embracing a healthier lifestyle, but the real journey unfolds with each day that comes.

Remember, your path to wellness is uniquely yours. It's a road paved with personal victories and challenges, moments of strength, and times of learning. There's no "one size fits all" regarding health; what matters most is finding what works for you, adapting, and continuing to move step by step.

Your journey doesn't stop here. Each day offers a new opportunity to make choices that support your health and well-being. Whether it's choosing nourishing foods, finding joy in movement, connecting with loved ones, or taking moments for self-care and reflection, these choices add up. They are the building blocks of a life lived well.

If you stumble or face obstacles along the way, remember that it's part of the process. These moments are not setbacks but stepping stones, opportunities to grow and learn. The path to wellness is not a straight line but a winding road with highs and lows. What's important is not how many times you might veer off the path but how many times you choose to get back on it.

You are not alone on this journey. Surround yourself with people who uplift and support you, and don't hesitate to reach out for professional guidance when you need it. There's strength in community and comfort in knowing that others are walking alongside you, each of us striving towards our own version of health and happiness.

As you move forward, carry the knowledge that your health is not just a series of numbers on a scale or data points on a chart. It's about how you feel, both inside and out. It's about living life fully, with vitality and joy. It's about being kind to yourself, celebrating your progress, and embracing each day with hope and determination.

Did you find value in the insights and guidance shared in this book? If so, I warmly encourage you to leave a **"positive review"** on Amazon. Your feedback is not just a support to others on a similar journey; it also amplifies our mission of promoting health equity and the significance of informed lifestyle decisions. Your voice can be a beacon for change, inspiring others to embark on their paths toward better health and happiness.

Thank you for your invaluable support and for contributing to this vital dialogue.

"Here's to your health, your journey, and the vibrant life that awaits you. May it be filled with joy, discovery, and wellness in every sense of the word."

Dr. Grace Totoe

About the Author

"Dr. Grace Totoe"

Meet Dr. Grace Totoe, a compassionate physician, entrepreneur, and health equity advocate dedicated to making a difference in the world, one patient at a time. With an impressive career spanning healthcare and entrepreneurship, Dr. Totoe stands out as a beacon of hope and change, especially within minority communities.

As the medical director of the Minneapolis Health Clinic (https://minneapolishealthclinic.com/), Dr. Totoe leads a team of healthcare professionals committed to providing top-notch medical care. Her approach goes beyond treating symptoms, focusing on preventive care and lifestyle changes as the cornerstone of good health. She believes everyone deserves quality healthcare, regardless of background or circumstances.

But Dr. Totoe's passion doesn't stop at the clinic doors. She is the driving force behind the Totoe Health Equity Project, a nonprofit organization with a mission close to her heart. Through this project, Dr. Totoe works to promote health equity among minority communities, paying special attention to the needs of African immigrants. Her efforts aim to bridge the gap in healthcare disparities, providing education, resources, and support to those who need it most.

Her work is a testament to her belief that health is a right, not a privilege. Dr. Totoe's commitment to health equity is not just about addressing immediate healthcare needs; it's about creating a sustainable model of care that empowers individuals and communities to take control of their health. Through her clinic and nonprofit, she offers a ray of hope, showing that it's possible to overcome the barriers to good health with the right support, education, and care.

Dr. Totoe's dedication to her patients and her community is unwavering. She embodies the values of compassion, innovation, and equity, making her a respected figure in healthcare and an inspiration to many. Whether she's in the clinic, leading her nonprofit, or sharing her knowledge and experiences, Dr. Totoe is driven by a simple yet powerful vision: a world where everyone, regardless of their background, has the opportunity to live a healthy, fulfilling life.

In writing this book, Dr. Totoe extends her mission beyond the walls of her clinic and the scope of her nonprofit. She invites readers on a journey towards better health, armed with the knowledge, strategies, and inspiration needed to make lasting changes. With Dr. Totoe as your guide, you're not just reading a book but taking a step toward a healthier future.

Essential Resources for Your Weight Loss Journey

As you continue your weight loss journey, having the right tools and resources can make all the difference in achieving your goals. To support you in this endeavor, I've compiled a list of recommended monitoring apps, sleep aids, exercise communities, meditation guides, and sources for more healthy recipes. These resources are designed to keep you informed, motivated, and on track towards a healthier lifestyle.

Monitoring Apps:

- **MyNetDiary:** Ideal for tracking nutrition and diet management, helping you stay aware of your eating habits.

- **MyFitnessPal:** A widely-used app for tracking nutrition and physical activity, providing a comprehensive view of your health journey.

- **Free Pedometers:** Various apps can transform your smartphone into a pedometer, making it easy to track your daily steps and stay active.

- **Oura Ring:** This innovative smart ring monitors your sleep patterns, daily activity levels, and overall health, offering insights into how you can improve your well-being.

Sleep Sounds on YouTube:

YouTube offers various sleep sound options for those who find solace in soothing background noises. Simply search "sleep sounds" on the platform to discover a variety of calming audio tracks designed to enhance your sleep quality.

Exercise Communities:

Fitbit Community, Nike Training Club, and Strava: These platforms offer a space to connect with like-minded fitness enthusiasts. Here, you can find support motivation and access free workout resources tailored to various interests and fitness levels.

Meditation Guides:

Headspace, Calm, and Insight Timer: These apps provide guided meditations to help reduce stress and improve mindfulness. For visual learners, YouTube hosts a plethora of meditation videos. Search terms like "guided meditation" or "meditation for beginners" can lead you to content that fits your needs and preferences.

Healthy Recipes:

To assist you in preparing nutritious meals that support your weight loss goals, consider exploring the following websites for inspiration:

https://www.eatingwell.com/gallery/7902553/weight-loss-recipes-for-beginners/

https://www.bbcgoodfood.com/recipes/collection/healthy-dinner-recipes-to-lose-weight

https://www.taste.com.au/healthy/galleries/healthy-dinner-ideas-weight-loss/6oetyh5j

By integrating these resources into your daily routine, you'll be well-equipped to navigate the challenges and successes of your weight loss journey. Remember, achieving your health goals involves small, consistent steps. With the right support and tools, you can make lasting changes that lead to a healthier, happier you.

Reference Resources (Materials)

https://www.ncbi.nlm.nih.gov/pmc/articles/PMC4229150/

https://www.who.int/news-room/fact-sheets/detail/obesity-and-overweight

https://www.hsph.harvard.edu/obesity-prevention-source/obesity-causes/physical-activity-and-obesity/#:~:text=Physical%20activity%20increases%20people's%20total,the%20development%20of%20abdominal%20obesity.

https://www.ncbi.nlm.nih.gov/pmc/articles/PMC3428710/#:~:text=Stress%20can%20also%20enhance%20weight,the%20rewarding%20properties%20of%20foods.

https://www.ncbi.nlm.nih.gov/pmc/articles/PMC5726407/

https://www.lifespan.org/lifespan-living/sleep-obesity-and-how-they-are-related#:~:text=Sleeping%20seven%20to%20eight%20hours,of%20becoming%20overweight%20or%20obese.

https://www.ncbi.nlm.nih.gov/pmc/articles/PMC4105579/

https://www.youtube.com/watch?v=zZhzjA968Xw

Made in the USA
Monee, IL
04 November 2024

69370188R00075